NTRAL
REGON

Walks,

Hikes &

Strolls

for
MATURE
FOLKS

2nd Edition

Marsha Johnson
Wendy Gray

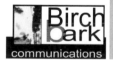
Birch bark
communications

Central Oregon
Walks, Hikes & Strolls for Mature Folks, Second Edition

Copyright © 2011, 2006, 2003, 2002 by Marsha Johnson

Published by
Birch Bark Communications
P O Box 129
Bend OR 97709

The authors express their appreciation to Bob Johnson, who hiked many miles with them and to the friendly personnel at Bend Metro Parks and Recreation and the Deschutes National Forest Service who provided useful information.

Cover Photos: Front – Three Creek Lake
Back – Sparks Lake

Printed in the USA by Maverick Publications, 2011, 2006, 2003, 2002
ISBN 0-9718996-1-4

For
Delbert and Betty Gray
who passed along
to us
their love
of the outdoors

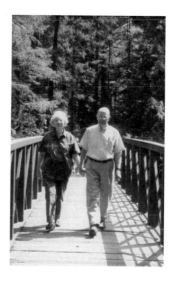

OUTING LOCATER

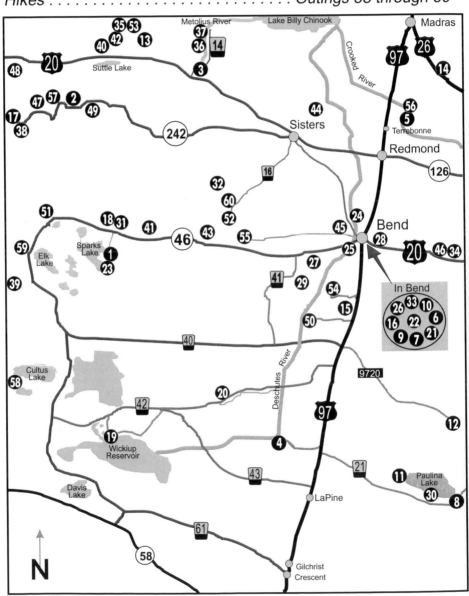

CONTENTS

CONTENTS

MEADOWS

31 Soda Creek Meadow
36 Metolius River North
41 Todd Lake
42 Canyon Creek Meadow
50 Benham Falls
51 Wickiup Plain
58 Muskrat Lake
60 Golden Lake

DESERT

14 Rimrock Springs
34 Horse Ridge Dry Canyon
44 Alder Springs
46 Badlands

WATERFALLS

11 Paulina Falls
17 Proxy Falls
18 Fall Creek Falls
29 Dillon Falls
32 Whychus Creek Falls
35 Wasco Lake
38 Linton Lake
42 Canyon Creek Meadow

RIVERS & STREAMS

3   Head of the Metolius
5   Smith Rock Viewpoint
7   Old Mill
11 Paulina Falls
13 Head of Jack Creek
15 Drake Park
17 Proxy Falls
18 Fall Creek Falls
20 Fall River
21 South Deschutes
22 First Street Rapids
24 Tumalo State Park
25 South Canyon Reach
26 Sawyer River Trail
27 Lava Island Falls
29 Dillon Falls
31 Soda Creek Meadow
33 South Canyon East
32 Whychus Creek Falls

THEME OUTINGS

36 Metolius River North
37 Metolius River South
38 Linton Lake
42 Canyon Creek Meadow
44 Alder Springs
45 Shevlin Park
50 Benham Falls
55 Tumalo Creek Canyon
56 Smith Rock
60 Golden Lake

more Rivers/Streams

ENCHANTING LAKES

1 Ray Atkeson Memorial
19 South Twin Lake
23 Sparks Lake
30 Paulina Lake
35 Wasco Lake
38 Linton Lake
39 Blow & Doris Lakes
40 Square Lake
41 Todd Lake
42 Canyon Creek Meadow
47 Tenas Lakes
48 Patjens Lakes
49 Matthieu Lakes
52 Tam McArthur Rim
53 Carl Lake
58 Muskrat Lake
59 Island Meadow
60 Golden Lake

PANORAMIC VISTAS

1 Ray Atekeson Memorial
2 Dee Wright Observatory
8 The Big Obsidian Flow
15 Lava Butte
23 Sparks Lake
26 Sawyer River Trail
28 Pilot Butte
30 Paulina Lake
41 Todd Lake
43 Tumalo Mountain
44 Alder Springs
46 Badlands

6

49 Matthieu Lakes
51 Wickiup Plain
52 Tam McArthur Rim
56 Smith Rock
57 Belknap Crater
60 Golden Lake

more Panoramic Vistas

FABULOUS FORESTS

13 Head of Jack Creek
29 Dillon Falls
31 Soda Creek Meadow
36 Metolius River North
38 Linton Lake
42 Canyon Creek Meadow
45 Shevlin Park
48 Patjens Lakes
49 Matthieu Lakes
50 Benham Falls
51 Wickiup Plain
58 Muskrat Lake

LAVA FLOW

1   Ray Atkeson Memorial
2   Dee Wright Observatory
8   Big Obsidian Flow
12 Lava Cast Forest
15 Lava Butte
17 Proxy Falls
23 Sparks Lake
27 Lava Island Falls
29 Dillon Falls
30 Paulina Lake
38 Linton Lake
49 Matthieu Lakes
50 Benham Falls
51 Wickiup Plain
54 Lost Forest
57 Belknap Crater

NO PASS REQUIRED

3   Head of the Metolius
4   The Big Tree
6   Juniper Park
7   Old Mill

9   Larkspur Trail   *more No Pass Required*
10 Ponderosa Trail
14 Rimrock Springs
16 Drake Park
20 Fall River
21 South Deschutes
22 First Street Rapids
25 South Canyon Reach
26 Sawyer River Trail
27 Lava Island Falls
28 Pilot Butte
33 South Canyon East
34 Horse Ridge Dry Canyon
36 Metolius River North
37 Metolius River South
44 Alder Springs
45 Shevlin Park
46 Badlands

CANYONS

5   Smith Rock Viewpoint
26 Sawyer River Trail
29 Dillon Falls
33 South Canyon East
34 Horse Ridge Dry Canyon
37 Metolius River South
44 Alder Springs
45 Shevlin Park
46 Badlands
50 Benham Falls
53 Carl Lake
55 Tumalo Creek Canyon

ACCESSIBLE

1   Ray Atkeson Memorial
2   Dee Wright Observatory
3   Head of the Metolius
4   The Big Tree
5   Smith Rock Viewpoint
7   Old Mill
11 Paulina Falls (to 1st viewpoint)
12 Lava Cast Forest
15 Lava Butte

INTRODUCTION

Initially written for seniors, *Walks, Hikes & Strolls for Mature Folks* has been well–received by Central Oregonians of all ages and fitness levels. There's an adventure here to please everyone, whether you want a strenuous mountain hike or a short, scenic side trip. In this Second Edition we've added ten new outings – three strolls, two walks and five hikes. The original outings have been updated (including updates in the 2011 printing) to reflect changes in our ever–changing area. It is our hope that this edition will provide many hours of enjoyment.

This guide addresses a wide range of senior needs and desires, as they relate to hiking and walking, with empathy and humor. It's not just for folks aged 65 and up but also for baby boomers like us, near the half–century mark, with an awakening understanding of "seniordom." We can't see as well or hear as well as we used to, and a number of body parts hurt more than they used to. Our knees and backs are a definite concern, and without ibuprofen and stretching, the back country would be off limits.

The number–one goal of our guide is to encourage and facilitate your enjoyment of the stunning beauty of our area. It aims to get you out of the recliner and into the wilderness where you can experience euphoric highs you might have thought were no longer possible. (Bonus: these highs are cheap and low–risk.) It includes a wide variety of outings, recognizing the wide range of abilities in our mostly over–fifty age group. Very fit baby boomers and seniors will find something here, as will those in wheelchairs. Some of the outings take groups into consideration, offering activity levels for all (see Appendix C).

We've had the privilege of visiting many of this country's mountain ranges and national forests, from the Smokies in Tennessee and the San Juans in Colorado to the Sawtooths in Idaho and the Sierras in California. Each area has its own magic and charm. But we've seen nothing in our travels to diminish our appreciation for Central Oregon, with its mountains, forests and deserts; streams, rivers and lakes; not to mention the largest variety of volcanic formations in the lower 48 states! How blessed we are to have access to such splendor!

FACTS

Central Oregon is home to open rangeland, a national grassland, over 2 million acres of national forest and eight wilderness areas. Several state parks and numerous city parks provide additional opportunities for outdoor recreation.

"You're only young once, but you can stay immature indefinitely."

Ogden Nash

TIDBITS

TIDBITS

The American Hiking Society claims that hiking regularly can reduce high blood pressure and cholesterol levels, lower the risk of heart disease, slow the aging process, improve osteoporosis and relieve back pain. It's also one of the leading ways to lose weight.

non omnia possumes omnes
(we cannot all do everything)

"Do not let what you cannot do interfere with what you can do."

John Wooden

The second goal of our book is to urge you to exercise (oops, there we've said it — the *e*–word). If motivation is a problem for you, consider the fact that after we pass age 30 or so, our metabolism starts slowing down by about 5% a year. We start losing muscle and bone mass. If we don't make a point of engaging in regular exercise, by the time we're 65 we can lose half our muscle mass and have our metabolism slow to burning 200–300 fewer calories a day. Any kind of exercise will help to counteract this progression by strengthening lean body mass, metabolism and immune response, and by maintaining stamina, strength, circulation and joint mobility. Walking is one of the easiest, safest and most rewarding ways to exercise! Cast aside your fear. Almost everyone can participate in at least one of the outings in this guide. Buck the national trend toward obesity and low fitness levels! Do something to raise your spirits! Soak in some natural beauty! Get out of that chair and take a walk!

Here's one further suggestion to motivate you to step out and enjoy the outdoors. Get into your car and drive to the Newberry National Volcanic Monument (fee site) south of Bend. Once in the park, drive up Paulina Peak to the overlook (accessible July–October). Wow, what an inspiring sight! Experience what Katherine Lee Bates must have felt when she penned *America the Beautiful* from atop Pikes Peak. Bask in the exhilaration of the pure air and the panoramic views. Imagine how much greater your exhilaration will be when you expend a little energy and attain a pristine mountain lake, a rarefied viewpoint or an old–growth forest where no vehicles can travel!

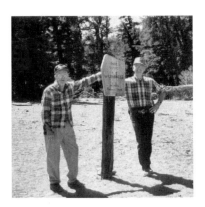

Part One

HITTING THE TRAIL

So you're considering the challenge of venturing out into our beautiful Central Oregon country **on foot**. A veritable banquet for the senses awaits you! You might need to invest some time and energy in preparing to go, but we can almost guarantee big dividends. The following pages offer tips and orientation information for the trail novice. They also include useful facts and interesting trivia for more seasoned hikers. It is our hope that mature folks will find encouragement to start walking, to keep walking, or perhaps to walk farther — for pure enjoyment and for better health.

THE MATURE HIKER

"One day some of the other teachers and I decided to go on a trip to 14,000-foot Pikes Peak. We hired a prairie wagon. Near the top we had to leave the wagon and go the rest of the way on mules. I was very tired. But when I saw the view, I felt great joy. All the wonder of America seemed displayed there, with the sea-like expanse."

Katherine Lee Bates, author of
America the Beautiful

Over the course of our adult lives our hiking habits have changed. As young people living in East Texas, the word *hike* was not in our vocabulary. We walked a trail on rare occasions, but swimming was our favorite activity. We did, however, develop a love of the woods from years of camping with our family. We learned what hiking is all about when we started spending time in Oregon and Colorado. After taking several backpacking trips and climbing a number of Colorado Fourteeners and Oregon Cascades, we felt we had earned our *hiker* status. A funny thing has happened, though, as we have aged and started hiking with other aging folks. We've developed a broader perspective — our own *mature hiker philosophy*. We no longer feel the need to keep up with the youngsters or to amass miles and peaks. We're less likely to compare or favor certain trails than to appreciate each for its uniqueness. We don't wear timer watches, and we're as apt to take a nap or meal at timberline as to pound on up to the peak. Yet still we are addicted to trekking through an enchanting forest, "discovering" a mountain tarn, and getting above treeline.

In recent years we've hiked with seniors and baby boomers of varying fitness levels. Our dad is fairly fit for his late seventies, a regular golfer but not a regular hiker. He loves forests and views and recently surprised himself by hiking up Tam McArthur Rim. Mom also enjoys forest outings, but with her osteoporosis she cannot risk falling; she needs smooth trails with very small changes in elevation. A friend loves hiking up mountains; her current health prevents an all–day climb, but she'll push herself for a couple of hours just to reach timberline on Broken Top. Another friend has a degenerative disease of the spine and walks with a cane, but her doctor has advised her to take short walks whenever she can. Then there's the couple in their seventies that Marsha and her husband ac-companied to a mountain lake in the Eagle Cap Wilderness. That trek was fourteen miles round trip with significant elevation gain. It was a challenge just to keep up with the seniors!

This guide recognizes that some of us still appreciate a physical challenge. The outings termed *HIKES* are for us. Within this category are mostly medium length (8 miles or less), medium elevation gain (800' or less), outings. A few longer and steeper hikes, with some extra challenges thrown in, are included for the adventurous.

The section on *WALKS* describes outings which are shorter than the hikes. Most don't have great elevation gains. These are for folks such as our dad, many of whom could manage some of the hikes, too. Then there are the *STROLLS*. These are suitable for our mom. They're mostly level with fairly smooth surfaces and even shorter distances than walks. A few of the strolls have paved, accessible paths that might be appropriate for folks in wheelchairs. Appendix C lists outings for groups with folks of varying fitness levels; included are two or more suggested treks or activities with a common staging area.

Before we proceed, let's say a word about these forty something to eighty–something persons we call *Mature Hikers*. Several characteristics set us apart from other (younger) hikers. First of all, to us, a Powerbar does not constitute a meal. Open–air outings mean fried chicken and potato salad! Fortunately, most of us have learned to compromise — chicken in a backpack is not pretty. Second, at almost any given time, something on our bodies either hurts or is not functioning optimally. And we usually think more in terms of coffee breaks (food), potty breaks (comfort), and bone breaks (caution), than how many lakes we can see or how much altitude we can gain in an outing. Lastly, we're not embarrassed to capitalize on our greater maturity and wisdom by slowing down and really enjoying the opportunity, which we no longer take for granted, to be out in the beautiful Central Oregon countryside.

Mobility is a gift! Enjoy it — treasure it — while you can!

Pre–planning, physical preparation *and* prudent mileage goals help alleviate most hiking complaints.

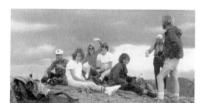

Senior hikers tend to voice the same complaints as younger hikers — blisters, aching muscles and knee problems.

WHAT TO KNOW BEFORE YOU GO

One of the best things about day hiking is that it's relatively inexpensive and uncomplicated. You don't need much more than comfortable walking shoes, a small pack and a water bottle. There are, however, tricks of the trade that will contribute to the success of these outings. We share with you here, and in the sections that follow, trail tips gleaned over our years of hiking in the region. More experienced hikers have permission to skip ahead.

Smart Going

Even when the weather is fine, the mature hiker should prepare for the unexpected. Accidents can happen to anyone, but we are perhaps a bit more susceptible than younger hikers. We suggest not going alone on an outing.

TRAIL ETIQUETTE: *Horseback riders* have the right of way. *Hikers & bikers*, move off the trail; don't make sudden movements or noise. *Bikers*, slow down when approaching *hikers*; give them plenty of room to pass.

■Tell someone *where you're going* and *when you'll return*. If you're planning to take one of the walks or hikes, it's a good idea to leave with someone a description of your vehicle and license number, your destination, and the names of people in your party.

■*Carry a cell phone.* While there are some places in the central Cascades where a cell phone is out of contact, having one along gives you an added measure of security. Keep in mind, however, that you may not be able to use it, depending on your location.

■Carry a *daypack or fanny pack* with the *essentials* we'll discuss below.

WHAT TO TAKE

The Cascades Mountaineers and other organizations recommend *ten essentials* a hiker should take on wilderness outings. While we certainly endorse this list and use it ourselves on some excursions, we realize that most outings in this guide are of the shorter, not so remote variety. Thus we recommend essentials based upon length and location of your outing.

Strolls

water bottle, sun protection

Walks

add daypack or fannypack, windbreaker/windpants, food, cell phone, T.P. (toilet paper), medications and small first–aid kit, mosquito repellent add space blanket or garbage bag, waterproof matches, extra food & water, whistle, map, pocket knife

Hikes

camera, binoculars, chapstick, guide book, compass, water purification tablets, small signal mirror, flashlight, thermos of espresso, 5–course meal, the butler and a llama to pack it all

Nice to Have

More About Gear & Essentials

Footwear

Well–fitting, stable walking shoes are the most important item for the enjoyment of your walk. Comfort is the key word here, and what's comfortable to you is what you should wear. No walk or hike is enjoyable if your feet are speaking to you. The best hikes are those during which you give no thought at all to your feet. You may find after hiking several trails that your needs will change. Some will prefer hiking boots for better support, but they're not necessary for most of the outings in this guide. Marsha loves her Montrail boots for their roomy comfort and sturdy support. Wendy has hiked in Vasque Sundowners for over twenty years, and while pricey, the Gore-tex–lined leather boot fits her foot like a glove. They've crossed many creeks and snowfields, provided stability on scree and cushioning on lava, and kept her dry and blister–free.

> Happy feet make for an enjoyable hike!

If you do decide to purchase new boots, try them on in the afternoon when your feet are most swollen to ensure an accurate fit. Also, we suggest you buy one–half size larger than your street shoes, to allow for wool socks and downhill stretches when your toes slide forward. They should be large enough to allow your toes to wiggle, but snug in the heel.

> Americans spend an average of $920 million annually on hiking boots, buying enough boots to stretch from Seattle to Buenos Aires.

Pack

Whether you choose to carry a daypack or a fanny pack, comfort is the key. If you are purchasing a pack for the first time, load it, try it on and wear it around the store, adjusting the straps to find a comfortable fit. Look for one with padded shoulder straps (or hip straps), and a padded back for extra comfort. Durable, weatherproof fabric and storm flaps over the zippers will keep contents dry. The only other requirement is that it have room for the essentials already mentioned. Fanny packs today come in sizes plenty large enough for the necessary items. We like a pack with two side pockets, one to hold a camera and the other for a water bottle, so each of these items is easily accessed without taking off the pack.

Food

You'll never find us without it! Pack for length of trip (plus extra for emergencies), and convenience weighed against comfort. A club sandwich is much more comforting than a meal bar, but bars are compact and impervious to jostling. We often take a bagel, some cheese sticks, fruit, several granola bars, and a couple meal bars for emergencies. Marsha's favorite bar is Bodhi Bar, available at health food stores (no refined sweeteners, low fat, no dairy or wheat, plus ginseng for energy). Wendy's favorite bar is chocolate, available everywhere (refined sugars, dairy, plus calories for energy). *CAUTION: some bars are hard to chew!*

> You'll burn 4 – 6 calories per minute when you walk 2 – 4 miles per hour.
> You'll burn 6 – 8 CPM walking 5 MPH.

Water

You need more water than you think; take at least a quart, and on longer hikes, take extra. As mature folks, we need hydration more than the twenty–somethings. Age causes our bodies to dehydrate more quickly. Water, the old–fashioned health drink, acts as a natural lubricant to limbs and joints, as well as keeping you more mentally alert. It is essential for *every* bodily process. Always carry more water than you think you will need, and always drink before you get thirsty. Staying hydrated and staying dry are the two most important things for seniors in the wilderness. *Note: do not drink water from backcountry streams and lakes.*

> Fitness experts advise drinking 16 ounces of water before an outing and 5 ounces every 20–30 minutes while walking.

Cell Phone

If you have a cell phone, take it with you, shut off in your pack, but available to use if needed. Although the Cascade Mountaineers claim that there are very few places in the Central Cascades wilderness areas where a cell phone is out of contact, we have had varying success when we've tried to use one in remote or mountainous terrain. Nevertheless, having one along certainly gives you the option of trying and possibly being able to use it.

These are optional, but we've found that they can turn a tentative hiker into a more confident hiker. We often hike with one pole each. It's great for creek crossings and steeper trails. If you have ski poles, you can buy rubber tips that convert them to trekking poles. The advantage of actual trekking poles is that you can telescope them, making them very short for stashing in your pack, longer for going downhill, shorter for going uphill. We used to be a little skeptical about the need for poles, thinking it just another opportunity to spend money on high tech gear that's really unnecessary. But then we hiked with a friend's poles and found that they really did help in several ways on steeper and rougher walks. The poles with shock–absorbing springs take stress off your joints, especially on downhill sections; every small advantage or comfort is significant at our age.

Trekking Poles

Hiking sticks have been around since the middle ages and earlier. The new trekking poles enhance the hiking experience, providing balance and taking stress off the knees.

As in the case of footwear, comfort is the key. A windbreaker and windpants of some type are essential. If you're hiking on a warm summer day, you'll probably start out in a tee–shirt and shorts, but the sweat of exertion can cause a chill once you reach higher elevations; you'll be glad you have a windbreaker along when you stop for lunch at a high mountain lake. Also keep in mind that, while rare in Central Oregon, the occasional rain shower may surprise you; staying dry is important for seniors, who tend to lose body heat more rapidly than younger folks.

Outerwear

Another essential garment for the mature rambler is headwear of some type. Put delicately, most of us, both male and female, do not have as much between our scalp and the sun as we once did; it's important to protect that tender body part from direct exposure. And don't be fooled by cloudy days either — remember that the sun is always there, doing what it does, toasting your head, face and eyes. There are unlimited numbers of headwear options, but if you're purchasing new headwear for your outings, we suggest you get something that provides UV protection for your face, ears, nose, eyes, and neck. Sunday

Headwear

Afternoons has a Derma-Safe line of headwear (SPF 30) that blocks UVA and UVB rays for dermatology patients dealing with skin cancer, melanoma, lupus, chemotherapy, cosmetic surgery, burns, and balding or hair loss. You can find their products at www.sundayafternoons.com.

Otherwear

If hiking gets into your blood, you will probably want to invest in a few other items for comfort. Wool socks (such as Smartwool Socks) or synthetic socks (look for Dupont Coolmax fiber) will wick moisture away from your feet and help prevent blisters. Shirts made of Coolmax or Techwear also wick moisture and keep your upper body more comfortable. We've often used 100% silk undershirts. In cooler weather, the 100% silk long underwear pants are warm and comfortable, adding hardly any bulk under your outerwear. These are available at outdoor stores or mail–order stores such as L.L. Bean and Eddie Bauer. Outdoor stores also carry shorts and pants in newer blend fabrics that dry quickly and don't "swish" too badly.

Sun Protection

> Sunscreen and sunglasses are imperative. Hats are also helpful.

While proper headwear will provide most of your protection, we've found that sunglasses are usually needed as well, especially when hiking around water or snow or at higher altitudes. Eye protection is essential for more mature eyes (as you'll appreciate if your eyes have been sunburned). Glare off of water or snow can burn your eyes well before you feel dis-comfort; wear sunglasses with good UV protection in addition to your headwear. Sunscreen is necessary for all of us, but even more so as we age and our skin becomes more fragile. Never leave home without your sunscreen liberally applied.

Insect Repellent

If you've ever been out on the trail during mosquito season without some bug juice, you'll know what we mean when we say "don't leave home without it." Mosquitoes can ruin a lovely outing if you're unprepared. We like to use Avon's Skin So soft because it does not contain DEET, which is the active ingredient in most insect repellents. DEET is by far the most effective, but it can strip the coating off your Gore-tex, so it makes you wonder what it might do to your skin, not to mention your insides. Use DEET sparingly if you must; if possible stick with non–toxic products from the health food store or Skin So Soft, which works pretty well most of the time and is also effective against blackflies. You can always slip on your windpants and windbreaker for extra protection if you need it. A citronella candle or two may help around your picnic area for a short time. A hat with a brim keeps bugs away from your face, since many insects fly in an up–and–down pattern. If you know where mosquitoes hang out, you can avoid them during the worst part of the season. Take your breaks away from water or wetter areas. Windy passes are not as likely to be swarming with bugs as lush, grassy meadows or lakes. Mid–summer is mosquito season in our region; they usually disappear by late summer.

> **NOTE**
> *If you take one of the outings in this guide in* **mid–summer**, *you will likely encounter* **mosquitoes**.

Many seniors take regular medications. Always tuck in the medicines you take regularly, just in case you are stranded or out longer than expected. It goes without saying that this is especially important for diabetics and heart patients. We also carry along some ibuprofen and a Benadryl tablet (for unexpected allergic reactions).

Medications

HOW TO PREPARE

If you are already a regular hiker, you should have no problem with most of the excursions in this guide. None of the hikes involves technical climbing, although some do have a few breathtaking ups and downs. If you are not particularly fit, you can nevertheless enjoy many of the outings described here; just remember to not overdo. Start with easy walks and work up to harder, longer ones. *If you are just beginning to walk or hike, it is important to get medical clearance; it's even more essential for hikers with medical conditions common to older folks, such as cardiac and back conditions, osteoporosis, or diabetes, to seek doctor approval.*

Fitness

Be sure to get *medical clearance* before enjoying these outings.

Stretching

Preparation prevents problems! Get medical clearance! *Stretch!* Start slowly & build in intensity and length!

Stretching is a must for us. We do it before and after hiking. Stretching improves circulation and decreases build–up of lactic acid, the chemical that causes sore muscles. It also alleviates stiffness and prevents muscle strain so you can walk farther more comfortably and with less chance of injury. Before and after your hike, allow a few minutes for simple stretching movements of the hamstrings, quadriceps, calves, achilles tendons and shins. A good library book might supply adequate stretches for you; a physical therapist can customize a routine for your body's needs.

Dream Cream

We use MSM lotion liberally. It seems to help with muscle soreness and joint pain. MSM lotion comes in several different brands available at health food stores; be sure to check the label and get only what has 15% or more MSM. The brand called Blue Stuff or Super Blue Stuff contains emu oil and a higher percentage of MSM. It is available at www.bluespringwellness.com. Great stuff!

A WORD ABOUT. . .

Walking Well

Walk at a rate that's comfortable for YOU.

Ignore any pronouncements you may have heard about proper rates per mile or respectable elevation gains per hour. Whatever feels right to you is the right pace to walk. How fast you *can* hike is one thing; how fast you *want* to hike is another. If you are just beginning, remember that the goal of hiking is not penance. Only a comfortable pace can be sustained; plodders frequently arrive before dashers, who require frequent rest stops. We often deliberately dawdle along the first stretch of trail as a sort of warm–up. Once your body and limbs are warm, your pace will naturally pick up.

Pets

Keep your dog on a leash less than six feet long. On some trails in the national forests, dogs are not required to be on a leash but must be within 15 feet and under reliable physical or voice control at all times. This amount of control is difficult if your pet spots a squirrel; it's best to use the leash. Wildlife chasing is the most common cause of lost dogs. The volcanic cinders, lava, and pumice on some of the trails in this guide are capable of shredding your dog's soft paw pads. Consider not taking your dog along on these types of trails. Also remember that your dog will require plenty of water — you'll need to pack extra.

Mountain lions, or cougars, are seldom seen by humans; if you should happen to see a mountain lion, keep your distance. Do not turn your back — face the lion and back away slowly. Stay upright and make yourself appear as large as possible. American black bear also live in the back country of Central Oregon and can be very dangerous. Absolutely do not run if you spot a bear. Slowly back away and lift your arms to appear bigger. If he continues to follow you, stand your ground and yell, clap your hands and wave. While we won't see them in our region, Wendy once came face to face with a moose in Idaho's Sawtooth Mountains.

Wild Animals

DO NOT RUN if you see a bear or cougar. Face the animal and back away slowly.

If you see lightning, count until you hear the thunder. A ten second count means that lightning is two miles away. Go to a low area and avoid trees. Get away from other hikers — groups attract lightning. Get away from rocks, which hold less water than your body. Crouch down, knees and feet together. Crouching lessens your chances of becoming a lightning rod.

Lightning

Don't relieve yourself in the wilderness. Just kidding! Everyone has to relieve himself at one time or another while on the trail, some of us more often than others. The forest service has rules about this — basically, "bury or carry." Go 200 feet from trails, water, or campsites. Bury waste and carry out toilet paper; a zip lock bag works well. If you're not averse to outhouses, use those at the trailheads before you leave to lessen your chances of having to BIFF it on the trail. BIFFing (Bathroom In Forest Floor) is perfectly acceptable, but can present problems for less agile folks. But enough about this indelicate subject.

When Nature Calls

Car cloutings have become more and more common at trailhead parking lots. It takes just a few seconds for an experienced clouter to break into your vehicle and take everything of value in sight. Leave valuables at home or lock them in your trunk.

When we hike in the wilderness, we like to feel as if we are the first ones to discover a particular spot. When the DROPS (Dreaded Other People) leave signs of having been there, it can besmirch the experience for us. Respect the forest and the wilderness and those who come to enjoy it after you. Just remember how your own experience is enhanced when people ahead of you don't leave traces of their presence. Allow others the same sense of discovery that you've enjoyed by leaving rocks, plants, and other artifacts as you find them. And always remember, "Pack it in, pack it out."

HOW TO USE THIS GUIDE

Each of the outings in this guide has been selected

- for enjoyment of mature folks of varying fitness levels
- for proximity to Bend
- for interesting features - views, geology, water, forests, meadows
- because we have personally walked and enjoyed it

We've tried to provide information to help you select outings that are feasible for your fitness level. Each of the outings is narrated with trail notes from our own treks on the trails. Our hope is that by reading about each trek before you go, you'll be able to judge its appropriateness for yourself. The trail description section will also be helpful to read as you walk along, because it details specifics of the trail you'll not want to miss. The *Fact Finder* and *Feasibility Gauge* columns in the margins provide specific trail information to help you quickly assess the outing. For example, if you are a senior with osteoporosis, you might want to avoid a trail with lots of roots or loose rock to lessen your chance of a fall.

Fact Finder

The mileage from Bend to the trailhead.

Miles to Bend

We list the significant features in order of their prominence. These are *views, water* (lakes, falls, streams, or rivers), interesting *geology, forests, meadows* or *desert.* These are why you hit the trail.

Features

Detailed driving directions to the trailhead. Look also for the driving distance from Bend at the top of the page.

Getting There

Mileages may vary on some outings. When a mileage range is given, there are two choices of turnaround points for a shorter or longer walk.

Miles

Depending upon your physical condition, the elevation gain of a given trek will be more or less meaningful to you. Generally speaking, elevation gains of 100′ feet or less are not too taxing for even the most out–of–shape among us (excepting perhaps those folks with heart or respiratory conditions). Gains of 100′ feet or more begin to demand greater aerobic capacity and leg strength. Also keep in mind that descents of greater elevation gains can be somewhat hard on the knees if you're not used to walking downhill. (See Appendix D for suggestions.)

Elevation Gain

Required permits are listed here. The Northwest Forest Pass ($5/day, $30/year), is required to park at many of the forest trailheads; purchase at ranger stations and sports shops. Watch for changes; this system is under review. Purchase state park passes ($3/day) at self–serve stations in the parks. Free wilderness permits can be obtained and filled out at the wilderness trailheads, so we don't note them here.

Permit

Northwest Forest Pass
$5/day
$30/year
Purchase at ski and sports shops.

Check this feature before you go to be sure your destination trail is actually open. Some trails are open only during the summer months, while others remain open year round. Often trails are muddy from snow

Open

melt in spring and early summer, and dusty from hikers and horses in late summer. Sometimes the forest service relocates portions of trails to avoid downed trees or restoration areas. When heading for mountains or wilderness in June or July, call the forest service first to check on snow conditions (numbers in Appendix E).

> **Maps**

Trail maps and trailhead driving directions given with each outing should be adequate for most folks. This list provides you with the names of maps that may make your hiking experience more interesting, especially if you enjoy topographical maps that show elevation contours. The USGS maps can be purchased at outdoor and mapping stores or be downloaded from www.trails.com. The Deschutes National Forest Map, most recently published in July of 2001, is a good all–purpose map. The Geo-Graphics Wilderness maps are also excellent aids and are available, along with the Deschutes National Forest Map, at the Forest Headquarters in Bend or the Sisters Ranger District Headquarters in Sisters. *Please note that our listing of a map does not necessarily mean that the specific outing trail is marked on that map.*

USGS topo maps are listed; they give interesting details of the surrounding area but don't necessarily show the trail described in the outing.

Feasibility Gauge

> **Trail Condition**

Our own assessment, based on the last time we hiked the particular trail, will include concise descriptors: smooth, rocky, roots, gravel, woodchips, etc.

> **Trailhead Facilities**

Here we list any conveniences available at the trailhead, such as outhouses, picnic tables, Starbucks....

> **Exposure**

This indicates whether the trail is shady or open to the sun, or both.

> **Use**

Three icons indicate whether the trail is open to hikers, horses and mountain bikes. We also note the degree of use — light, moderate or heavy.

> **Notes**

We mention here any special problems or suggestions.

Part Two

STROLLS

From a short city saunter to a wild wilderness walk, the strolls are like party appetizers — some are hearty snacks and others just whet your appetite for something more. They tease you, and they prepare you for the other courses. Some of the strolls are actually desserts, treats that very fit hikers will want to indulge in. The outings in Bend are surprisingly enjoyable despite the urban setting, and there's no need to drive to a distant trailhead (thus eliminating one common excuse to stay on the couch). On the other hand, if you need an excuse to get out of town, the forest outings provide you with both a pleasant drive and pleasant physical activity.

FACT FINDER

Volcanic Oasis

28 miles to Bend

Geology
Water
View
Forest

Sparkling blue water, snow–capped mountains, and unique volcanic formations await you on this short barrier–free stroll. A favorite spot for internationally–known photographer Ray Atkeson, Sparks Lake will most likely become one of your favorite places, too. The paved path follows a gradual slope down to the lake overview. Some folks in wheelchairs might find it difficult to come back up the incline. We feel compelled to mention that the best outhouse in the Deschutes National Forest stands at this trailhead.

Getting there

- *Drive west from Bend 27 miles on Highway 46/Century Drive (go about 4 miles past Mt Bachelor Ski Resort).*
- *Turn left on Road 400 to Sparks Lake. Stay left for about 1 mile to a trailhead parking area near the boat landing.*

MILES
0.4

ELEV. GAIN
20'

PERMIT
NW Forest Pass

OPEN
July to October/ November

MAPS
Geo Graphics *Three Sisters Wilderness Map*, Deschutes National Forest Map, USGS *Broken Top*.

Locate the trailhead at the west end of the parking lot and turn right for this short and satisfying foray along the shores of Sparks Lake. Follow the smooth trail through a lodgepole pine forest where lava canyons and crevices give evidence of the area's volcanic history. A viewpoint provides benches for resting and enjoying the postcard vista across the lake to the Cascade snow caps. Look for lava shield volcanos, South Sister and Broken Top. Broken Top, with its eroded peaks, is thought to be extinct. South Sister, whose most recent eruption occurred 2000 years ago, is one of the region's most likely sites for future volcanic activity. It is being closely monitored by scientists since May, 2001, when an area of upward–swelling earth was detected west of the peak.

The paved path turns to dirt a short distance beyond the viewpoint. The longer loop trail is described in the *Walks* section of this guide (*Outing 23*). The return trip to the car retraces the paved trail; those in wheelchairs might appreciate assistance on the incline.

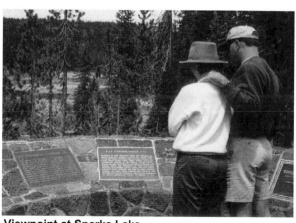

Viewpoint at Sparks Lake

TRAIL
CONDITION
paved

TRAILHEAD
FACILITIES
outhouse

EXPOSURE
airy forest

USE
🚶
moderate

♿

incline

STROLL

NOTES
*Mosquitoes likely
in mid-summer.*

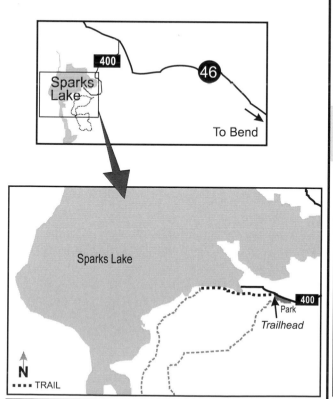

Sparks Lake

400

46

To Bend

Sparks Lake

400

Park
Trailhead

↑
N

▪▪▪▪ TRAIL

TIDBITS
Widely acclaimed
and widely exhi-
bited, Ray Atkeson
photographed the
scenic won-ders of
the West from the
1920's through the
1960's. In 1987,
Atkeson was named
Photographer Lau-
reate of the State of
Oregon.

FACT FINDER

36 miles to Bend

Geology View

As you stand on this 75–square–mile lava flow, imagine the difficulties confronting pioneer travelers over the summit. It is said that the early Scott party used as many as twenty–six oxen to haul one wagon up the steep, rocky grade. Walk the accessible path to learn more history of the area and to experience the unique geologic features and magnificent 360–degree views; you'll receive splendid returns for the small amount of time and effort invested!

Getting there

- *Drive west out of Sisters about 15 miles on the McKenzie Highway 242.*
- *Park on the south side of the highway at McKenzie Pass and walk across the road to the observatory.*

MILES
0.5

ELEV. GAIN
50'

PERMIT
NW Forest Pass

OPEN
July to October/ November

MAPS
Geo Graphics *Mt Washington Wilderness Map*, *Deschutes National Forest Map*, USGS *Mt Washington.*

The trail begins just east of the stairway to the observatory and winds through a centuries–old lava flow from Yapoah Crater to the south. Follow this lava river along sections of the Old Deschutes Wagon Road, constructed in the 1860's and 70's. Interpretive signs along the way explain the unusual formations. When you cross a lava "gutter," look left for views of Mt. Jefferson and Mt. Washington. At another "crack" in the flow, turn right and switchback up a slope through subalpine firs and whitebark pines to a U–turn that faces Black Crater. Next, pass through a mysterious canyon, wide then narrow, as you follow the trail back to the loop junction and on to the parking area. Take your time, or you'll miss the great variety in the rocks, spewed and cooled then flung to their resting spots in randomly artistic patterns.

While you're here, take advantage of the views from the quaint rock observatory named after well–known architect Dee Wright. Climb the staircase or use an accessible, gently–sloped path near the outhouse a few steps to the west. You'll see most of the Central Oregon Cascade snow caps from here, and you'll get a better perspective on the immensity of the lava flow. Belknap

Crater and Little Belknap Crater are prominent in the north foreground. Note the two tree "islands," or steptoes, that the lava bypassed as it flowed.

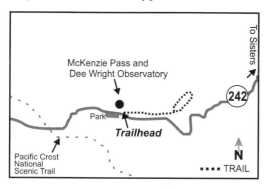

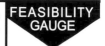

FEASIBILITY
GAUGE

TRAIL
CONDITION
paved

TRAILHEAD
FACILITIES
outhouse

EXPOSURE
open

USE
heavy

STROLL

View to the south from observatory

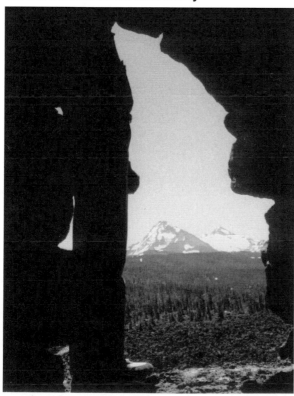

NOTES

Watch car traffic; stairs to climb to observatory.

TIDBITS

Sitting on lava flow from Yapoah Crater, the Dee Wright Observatory basalt blocks blend perfectly into the landscape, which has been called the "Black Wilderness." The younger Yapoah flow overlaps the older Belknap flow to the north. Felix Scott first drove cattle over this pass in 1860. A toll road was completed in 1872; the pass highway was paved in the 30's.

The Enchanted Waterway

35 miles
to
Bend

Water
Forest
View

"Picture perfect" just begins to describe this spot — perhaps you'll recognize it as the subject of a popular postcard. Our home in heaven may be built on a site such as this. Add the mystery of springs bubbling from rock to the serenity of a grassy meadow with tall trees, and throw in the grandeur of a snowy mountain backdrop; it just doesn't get much better on this planet! The stroll is short, but you'll want to allow extra time to bask in the beauty.

Getting there

- *Drive west from Sisters on Highway 20 almost 10 miles to a sign for Camp Sherman and the Metolius River.*
- *Turn right (north) on Road 14.*
- *Drive about 4 miles, staying right at a fork, to the parking area for Head of the Metolius.*

MILES
0.4

ELEV. GAIN
20'

PERMIT
none

OPEN
*April to
December*

MAPS
Deschutes National Forest Map, USGS ***Black Butte.***

Walk to the west side of the parking area to find the smooth path bordered by a rustic rail fence. Majestic ponderosa pine trees tower over manzanita, current and bunch grasses. The trail arrives shortly at an overlook with a good view of the river suddenly appearing under a rock bluff. The Metolius has its own unique set of vital statistics. Its consistent fifty–degree temperature and outstanding water quality provide a friendly habitat for the rare bull trout plus various other species of trout and salmon. Dropping about thirty–five feet per mile in a forty–one mile journey to Lake Billy Chinook, the clear, frigid river gains volume from the addition of several springs. It provides a recreation wonderland with opportunities to fish, camp, raft, kayak, hike, bike and picnic.

In addition to a good look at the headwaters, you'll enjoy the view across the meadowed bank to regal Mt. Jefferson, Oregon's second highest peak. Keep an eye out for deer and waterfowl. When you've gotten a sufficient dose of this remarkable loveliness, walk back up the trail, stopping at a bench if you need a rest.

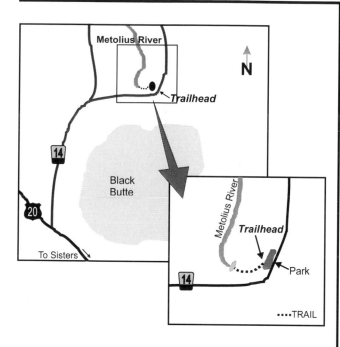

Metolius River

Trailhead

N

Black
Butte

To Sisters

Metolius River

Trailhead

Park

····TRAIL

FEASIBILITY
GAUGE

TRAIL
CONDITION
paved

TRAILHEAD
FACILITIES
*outhouse,
tables*

EXPOSURE
airy forest

USE

*moderate/
heavy*

NOTES
*Mosquitoes likely
in mid-summer.
Don't forget your
camera.*

TIDBITS

When Black Butte, a
volcanic cinder
cone, formed over
stream beds, wa-
ter backed up into a
swamp to the south
at present– day
Black Butte Ranch.
Some of the stream
water seeped
through porous
rocks to reappear as
the Metolius head-
waters.

Headwaters of the Metolius River

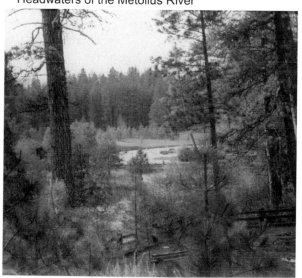

27 miles to Bend

Forest Water

The fun of this outing is in viewing a mammoth tree that's older than your great–great–great–great grandfather. You'll stand in awe of "Big Red," the national co–champion ponderosa pine. That it guards the banks of the picturesque Deschutes River, wide and peaceful here, is an added bonus.

Getting there

- *Drive south from Bend on Highway 97 about 22 miles.*
- *Turn right at a sign for LaPine State Recreation Area.*
- *Drive 4.3 miles and turn right at the sign for The Big Tree.*
- *Drive a short distance along a gravel road to a parking area.*

MILES
0.5 +

ELEV. GAIN
30'

PERMIT
none

OPEN
April to December

MAPS
Deschutes National Forest Map, USGS Pistol Butte.

The trail starts on the north side of the parking lot and heads northeast through a mixed pine forest to the venerable ponderosa and the Deschutes River just beyond. The famous pine, the largest in Oregon, is over 500 years old. It stands 165 feet tall and measures more than 8 feet in diameter. The other pines in the forest are youngsters by comparison. At some point in its long history, the big pine lost its upper trunk and branches, perhaps to a lightning strike. Frequent, light fires have contributed to the health of ponderosa forests. You'll notice here that the young trees have nearly black bark while mature trees are orange colored, giving rise to the nickname, "punkins." Very old trees have been called "yellow–bellies" because they appear almost golden in the sunlight.

Walk around the fenced area to the grassy river bank. This horseshoe bend in the Deschutes makes a good spot to picnic or explore. You can walk back the same way you came, or take the trail marked "Big Pine" near the river, which leads up a hill then back to your car on an old logging road littered with limbs (a bit treacherous for *Strollers*). The paved path from parking lot to the pine tree might be suitable for wheelchairs; it's probably too steep for some, and the last time we visited, there were numerous cracks along the way.

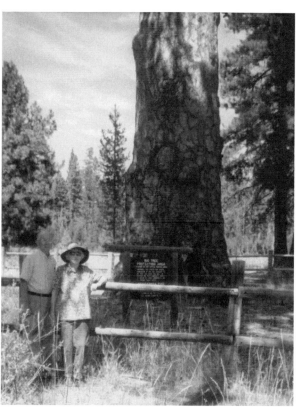

The Big Tree ponderosa pine

TRAIL
CONDITION
paved,
with cracks

TRAILHEAD
FACILITIES
outhouse

EXPOSURE
shaded

USE
🚶
moderate

♿

possibly

NOTES
Trekking poles
helpful for in-
clined path.

STROLL

TIDBITS

Half the trees east
of the Cascade
summit in Oregon
are ponderosa
pines. They thrive
on 15 or less
inches of annual
rain and live long
lives (one Oregon
tree lived to 726
years). The lum-
ber is prized for
many uses inc-
luding furniture,
residential con-
struction, toys and
crates.

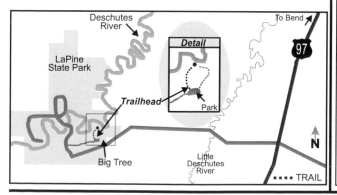

FACT FINDER

26 miles to Bend

Geology
Water
View

Smith Rock State Park provides a feast to the eyes for anyone who can get into a car and drive a few miles. Without ever leaving the vehicle, you can take in views of many of the park's extraordinary formations. If you don't mind descending to the river, you can create your own outing by walking in either direction as far as you choose. Here we've described a short, barrier–free trek along the canyon rim that affords wonderful cliff views and lets you watch climbers on Morning Glory Wall. You'll want your camera and binoculars.

Getting there

- *Drive north from Bend on Highway 97 through Redmond, then 5.4 miles beyond Redmond's north Y to Terrebonne.*
- *Turn right (east) on Wilcox Way and drive 2.6 miles to Crooked River Way.*
- *Turn left and drive 0 .7 miles to Smith Rock State Park.*
- *Purchase the parking permit near the information board and place on car dashboard.*

MILES
0.5 +

ELEV. GAIN
< 30'

PERMIT
state park pass

OPEN
all year

MAPS
Pick up trail map at Info Board.
USGS *O'Neil.*

At the south end of the main parking area, look for a crushed rock trail leading west. The path is barrier–free and should work for most wheelchairs with pneumatic tires. As you meander through sagebrush and juniper trees charred in a recent fire, watch for Cascade views beyond the cliffs. When you reach the main viewpoint with benches, stop to observe the rock climbers on the cliff faces across the Crooked River. Smith Rock State Park has gained fame in the last decade as a premier climbing destination. As home to one of the world's three most difficult routes, the park attracts top international climbers. Weekends are especially busy, but one can see climbers on almost any day when it's dry and the temperature exceeds forty degrees.

For a one–half mile stroll, walk back on the same path to the parking area. For a bit more exercise, continue along the trail to the walk–in camping area to the south. On the way, another viewpoint provides additional river views. A side trail leads west down to the river; however, most *Strollers* will not want to tackle this steep path. To return to your car from the camping area, go back the way you came (recommended), or take a path to the east and walk through a parking lot to rejoin the main trail before it reaches the street–side parking area.

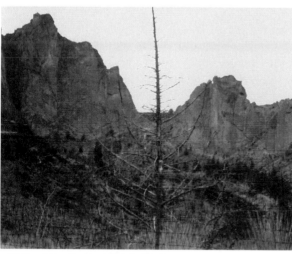

Cliffs at Smith Rock State Park

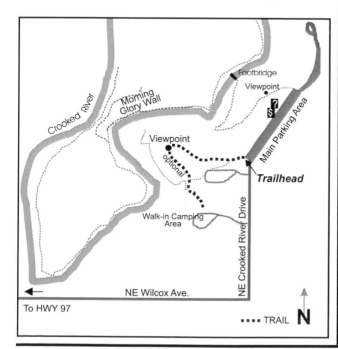

FEASIBILITY
GAUGE

TRAIL
CONDITION
*smooth,
crushed rock*

TRAILHEAD
FACILITIES
*pit toilets,
tables*

EXPOSURE
open

USE
🚶🚴
heavy

♿
pneumatic tires

STROLL

NOTES
Bring binoculars. Many additional walking options.

TIDBITS

A mecca for rock climbers, Smith Rock State Park claims several thousand climbs, with more than a thousand bolted routes.

IN
Bend

Occupying a full six blocks, Juniper Park provides a variety of activities for local residents and visitors. Facilities include tennis courts, horseshoe pits, a children's playground, a baseball field, and a renovated aquatic center with several swimming pools. The spongy walking trail is easy on the legs and it affords glimpses of the various activities as well as quieter moments under the junipers and pines.

Trees

Getting there

- *At the intersection of Business Highway 97 (Third Street) and Franklin Avenue, turn east and drive 0.4 miles to NE th Seventh Street.*
- *Turn left (north) into a parking lot adjacent to the Juniper Park tennis courts.*

MILES
0.9

ELEV. GAIN
< 30'

Find the paver path leading to the Aquatic Center, but turn left and walk west along a sidewalk, then continue up a slight hill between maintenance and restroom buildings. Curve to the right around the outdoor activity pool; fork left on the woodchip path and move past the playground to skirt the park's perimeter, turning north along NE Fifth Street. At the next fork, stay right and walk toward the pool, which was enlarged in 2006 to meet growing community demand.

PERMIT
none

Walk back to the starting point and look for the chip path near the tennis courts. Continue on the east loop trail, which curves east then west around a shady knoll with conifers and aspens. The path snakes around and for a short distance parallels NE Eighth Street, the park's eastern boundary.

OPEN
all year

Juniper Park is a grass–carpeted oasis populated by western juniper and ponderosa pine trees. Several rocky knolls contain native vegetation including Oregon grape. The park has served generations of Bendites. When our kids were small, they had fun searching for an obscure sign tacked to a ponderosa

MAPS
Bend City Map,
USGS *Bend.*

pine that held Joyce Kilmer's well–known words, "I think that I shall never see a poem lovely as a tree...." The trail makes a U–turn near Franklin Street then shortly delivers you back to your starting point.

Aquatic Center entrance

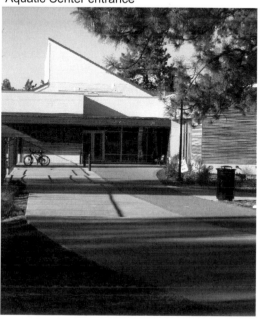

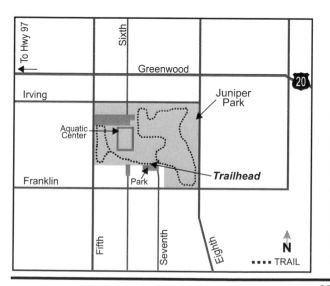

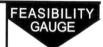

IN

Bend

The timber industry looms large in Bend history; the first commercial sawmill began operation in 1903. 1916 was the year of completion for the two large mills located at the site of this outing. The Shevlin–Hixon mill sawed its first log in March of that year, and the Brooks Scanlon Lumber Company began cutting in April. As you enjoy this stroll, try to imagine the bustling waterfront where horses moved lumber until 1958.

Water View

Getting there

- *From the intersection of Hwy 97 (Bend Parkway) and SW Colorado Avenue, drive west on Colorado 0.7 mile.*
- *Turn left on Industrial Way and follow the curve onto Bond Street, driving 0.4 miles to Powerhouse Drive.*
- *Turn right, drive a short distance and find a parking place in the Old Mill shopping district.*

MILES
1

ELEV. GAIN
negligible

PERMIT
none

OPEN
all year

To find the starting point for this outing, look for a unique sculpture near the Gap shop. Walk over the footbridge to cross the Deschutes River. Turn right and follow along the river, then turn left and skirt the edge of a the Les Schwab Ampitheater, noting views ahead of Tam McArthur Rim, Broken Top and South Sister. Make a left turn on a sidewalk along SW Shevlin Hixon Drive, and another on SW Columbia. After you re–cross the Deschutes, turn left on NW Theater, then left again to find the paved path along the river. Look for Mt. Bachelor and Tumalo Mountain to the west. Continue north behind the shops and past the footbridge. Walk to the east around a tiered pond, then to right along a sidewalk and right on Powerhouse Drive, so named for the three brick buildings nearby that housed boilers for generating steam to run the mill's giant saws. These powerhouses and the shiny refurbished smokestacks preserve a small piece of Bend's early history. As you return to your starting point, watch for several other relics from the timber heyday.

The Old Mill District affords numerous walking opportunities. Just upriver from the shops is Farewell

MAPS
Bend City Map,
USGS *Bend.*

Bend Park, which combines with Riverbend Park to make a 39 acre greenbelt. The two parks are connected by a footbridge over the Deschutes. This calm stretch of the river has become popular for floating on hot summer days. On some August afternoons, you'll see numerous sun–seekers in rafts and inner tubes. Continuing west through Farewell Bend Park takes you past a small swimming beach and under the car bridge to the trailhead for the South Canyon East trail (*outing 33* in this book).

Strolling among the shops provides pleasant exercise plus the opportunity to shop, eat or see a movie. *Warning: this outing can be hazardous to credit cards!*

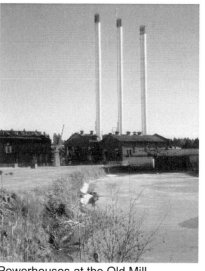
Powerhouses at the Old Mill

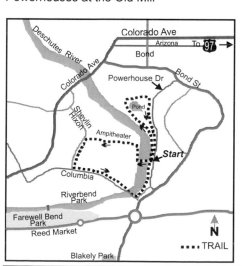

TIDBITS

Bend received its name from the large hairpin curve in the river here. At this location in 1877, John Y. Todd established his Farewell Bend Ranch, so named because pio-neers traveling the stage road enjoyed their last glimpse of the Deschutes at this bend.

A Fiery Past

**38 miles
to
Bend**

**Geology
View**

Established in 1990, the Newberry National Volcanic Monument encompasses 50,000 acres of geologic wonderland. The interpretive trail through a portion of the Big Obsidian Flow gives *Strollers* access to the grandeur of the area. Those who are challenged by the elevation gain may stop at the Lost Lake viewpoint. While you're in the park, try to visit Paulina Falls (see page 46) and Paulina Peak for further glimpses of unique volcanic features.

Getting there

- *Drive south from Bend 23 miles on Hwy. 97 to a sign for Newberry Caldera.*
- *Turn left (east) on Road 21 and drive 13 miles. At the entrance booth, purchase a NW Forest Pass if you don't have one.*
- *Continue driving 1.8 miles and turn right into the parking lot for the Big Obsidian Flow.*

**MILES
0.8**

**ELEV. GAIN
140'**

**PERMIT
NW Forest Pass**

**OPEN
June to
November/
December**

**MAPS
Deschutes National Forest Map,
USGS East Lake.**

Walk on the paved trail through an airy lodgepole pine forest to a metal staircase. Climb to a view of otherworldly Lost Lake, which lies between the forest and the steep face of the lava flow. Continue along the relatively smooth path to a bridge over a deep crack in the flow. A 0.4 mile loop leads to an overlook with views of Paulina Peak, the rim of Newberry Crater, East Lake, and Paulina Lake. With a depth of 250 feet, Paulina Lake is one of the deepest in the state. Interpretive signs along the trail will enlighten you with facts about the geologic history of the Big Obsidian Flow, considered to be one of the finest examples of obsidian flow in the world. At 1300 years old, this is also the youngest lava flow in Oregon.

As you walk back across the bridge toward the staircase, notice three types of rock: shiny, black obsidian glass; airy, gray pumice; and white pumice, with its numerous small holes. You may also see layered rocks composed of obsidian and pumice, both of which started as rhyolite magma. The glassy obsidian formed when the magma erupted without absorbing water, while bubbly pumice resulted from water absorption as the magma reached the surface. Take care when touching these sharp rocks, and be sure to leave them here; the park service prohibits collecting souvenirs.

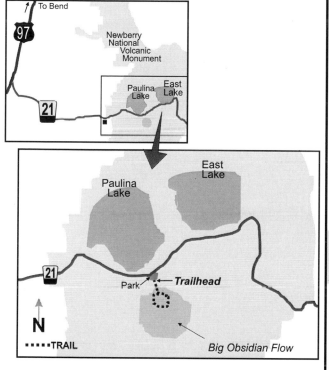

Lost Lake & Obsidian Flow

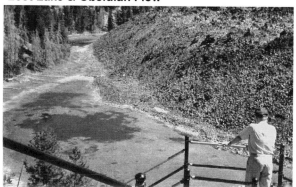

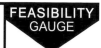

IN
Bend

The Larkspur Neighborhood Trail provides an easy way to get a little exercise within the city limits. Mature trees and a canal, some undeveloped land and a small airstrip contribute to the charming variety of the outing. *Strollers* will appreciate the smooth trail and the lovely new park with opportunities for picnicking and more walking. Children may want to try out the accessible play equipment. Adults should take a quick peek inside the Bend Senior Center.

Water
Trees

Getting there

- *Drive south on Business 97.*
- *Turn left on Reed Market Road and drive 1.1 miles. (Alternately, exit Hwy 97 onto Reed Market to the east. Cross Business 97 and drive 1.1 miles.)*
- *Turn left at the sign for Bend Senior Center.*
- *Park on the north side of the parking lot.*
- *Look for the trail near the Dog-E Rest Stop and a small bridge over a canal.*

MILES
1 +

ELEV. GAIN
negligible

PERMIT
none

OPEN
all year

MAPS
Bend City Map,
USGS *Bend.*

You'll find a trailmarker on a post near the Dog–E Rest Stop. The trail heads north along a small irrigation canal, a spur off the Central Oregon Canal. You'll walk on a combination of gravel and dirt surfaces sometimes quite near to houses but usually farther away. This path has a woodsy feel because of the many large ponderosa pines growing along the waterway. At times you can almost imagine yourself being far from town. Water runs in the canal from mid–April to mid–October. In spring and summer you might see baby ducks following in mother's wake. Cross the Bronzewood cul–de–sac and continue on the trail

After about one–half mile, you'll be surprised to see a short, paved airstrip tucked into a housing area. A sign designates this as Pilot Butte Airport. It's a private runway used by some of the homeowners — if you're really lucky, you might witness a landing or take–off. This is a good turnaround point for a one–mile walk. If you want to go farther, continue north behind homes that border the airstrip. When you come to Tempest

Drive, you can turn around or cross and continue on to Bear Creek Road, about one–half mile. (For an even longer outing, walkwest along Bear Creek and pick up the trail to the north which connects through the Highway 20 pedestrian underpass to Pilot Butte and its summit trail.)

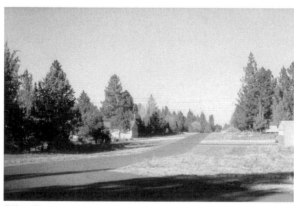

Pilot Butte Airstrip

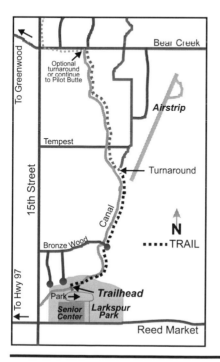

FEASIBILITY GAUGE

TRAIL CONDITION
smooth, gravel/dirt

TRAILHEAD FACILITIES
restrooms nearby in park

EXPOSURE
mostly shaded

USE

light

NOTES

One street crossing in a low-traffic area.

TIDBITS

The Bend Senior Center, which opened in fall of 2001, promotes active lifestyles for persons age 50 and up. Recreation programs and continuing education classes are offered as well as meals and social activities. The center's hours of operation are 8 am to 10 pm everyday.

STROLL

FACT FINDER

Serpentine Calorie Burner

IN
Bend

Leave your boredom at home and enjoy a trail that provides glimpses into Bend daily life: mountain views, youth playing at team sports, skateboarders, sounds of traffic and the prominence of Bend landmark, Pilot Butte. Burn off breakfast with no fuss and no long drive. You'll also have an opportunity to study typical high desert vegetation as you stroll along a smooth, level path.

View

Getting there

- *Drive east through Bend on Greenwood Avenue/Hwy 20E.*
- *Turn south (right) on SE Fifteenth Street at a traffic light on the south side of Pilot Butte.*
- *Drive about one-quarter mile beyond the traffic circle at 15th and Bear Creek and turn right into a parking lot at the north end of Ponderosa Park.*

MILES
1

ELEV. GAIN
30'

PERMIT
none

OPEN
all year

MAPS
Bend City Map,
USGS *Bend.*

Walk past the restrooms at the west end of the parking area and look for a blue trail marker sign on a pole. Walk south (clockwise on the loop) up a small rise on the woodchip path. In a very short distance the trail turns to grass and skirts around a rock wall edging a baseball field. Soon after you walk back into the brush, you'll come to a fork. Stay to the left, unless you prefer a very short stroll; if so, turn right. Continue walking on the woodchip, rock–bordered path, even though several dirt paths tempt you to stray. The trail snakes around like the Little Deschutes River, packing as many calorie–burning steps into the perimeter of the park as possible. Watch for glimpses of Mt. Bachelor, Tumalo Mountain, Broken Top, and South Sister. You'll also have good views of Pilot Butte. The Central Oregon "brush trio" is prevalent here — sagebrush, bitterbrush and rabbit brush— and you'll see ponderosa pines and western junipers. Just before reaching the starting point, the trail winds past a skateboard park. Pause a minute to watch the skaters. They may look a bit like aliens, but most of them are actually pretty nice folks out for some fresh air and exercise just as you are. Oh, to still have that kind of agility!

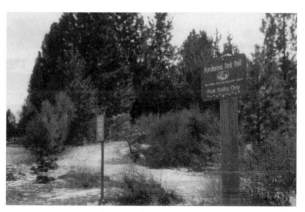

Trailhead in Ponderosa Park

FEASIBILITY
GAUGE

TRAIL
CONDITION
*smooth,
woodchip*

TRAILHEAD
FACILITIES
restroom

EXPOSURE
open

USE
🚶
moderate

STROLL

NOTES

Parking lot is very crowded some afternoons and evenings.

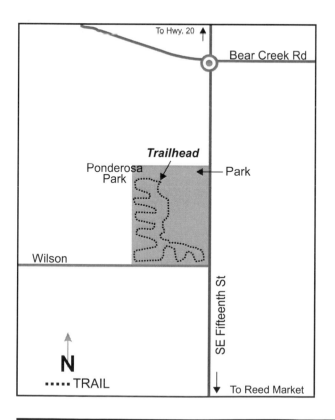

TIDBITS

The Bend Metro Parks and Recreation District maintains over 2,370 acres of parkland, 74 parks and 56 miles of trails. The BMPRD system is recognized throughout the Pacific Northwest as one of the best.

36 miles to Bend

Water
Forest
Geology

Paulina Falls is just one of an impressive list of worthwhile destinations in Newberry National Volcanic Monument (see also *outings 8, 12 and 30*). The only stream on Newberry Volcano, Paulina Creek flows through a gap in the 1000–foot walls of the caldera rim and thunders over a high ledge a short distance later. For this outing you can expend just a little energy or burn off most of lunch. The majestic waterfall is visible from three viewpoints; if you visit all three, you'll walk just under 1.7 miles. Even the short jaunt to the first overlook will reward you with the exhilaration of being near the deafening spray.

Getting there

- *Drive south from Bend 23 miles on Highway 97 to a sign for Newberry Caldera.*
- *Turn left (east) on Road 21 and drive 12.5 miles.*
- *Stop at the entrance booth to purchase a Northwest Forest Pass (day and annual passes available).*
- *Turn left into the parking loop for the falls.*

MILES
0.4 – 1.7

ELEV. GAIN
10 – 300'

PERMIT
NW Forest Pass

OPEN
June to November/ December

MAPS
Deschutes National Forest Map,
USGS *East Lake.*

You'll find the trailhead at the northeast end of the parking loop. Walk about fifty feet and turn right, continuing the short distance to the first viewpoint above Paulina Creek. A massive basalt cliff protrudes enough to split the creek into a double falls spilling onto the boulders below.

The second viewpoint can be reached by walking another one–half mile through the forest of lodgepole and ponderosa pines, subalpine firs and mountain hemlocks. The trail intersects a paved road leading into the caldera containing Paulina Lake. Walk over the bridge, turn left and continue down a dirt path parallel to the stream. The fenced overlook provides a good view of the smaller cascade.

To visit the third viewpoint, walk back to the junction near the parking area. Keep to the right and follow the relatively smooth trail as it snakes down to Paulina Creek. From this vantage point you'll enjoy the dramatic effect of the stream dropping over the 80–foot cliff in its two separate cascades. Return to the junction and turn right to arrive back at your car.

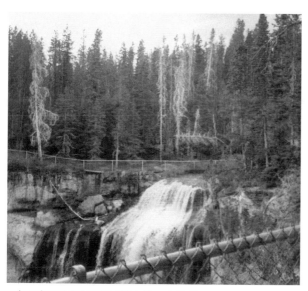

1st viewpoint at Paulina Creek Falls

TRAIL
CONDITION
mostly smooth

TRAILHEAD
FACILITIES
*outhouse,
tables*

EXPOSURE
shaded

USE
moderate

*to 1st
viewpoint*

STROLL

NOTES
*Trekking poles
helpful for descent
to creek.*

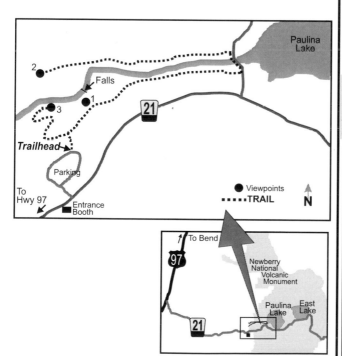

Paulina
Lake

Falls

2

3

1

21

Trailhead

Parking

To
Hwy 97

Entrance
Booth

Viewpoints
•••••TRAIL
N

To Bend

97

Newberry
National
Volcanic
Monument

Paulina   East
Lake   Lake

21

TIDBITS

Paulina Lake, at
250' deep, is home
to a large
population of trout
and salmon.
Paulina Creek
travels about 12
miles from the lake
to the Little
Deschutes River.
The Newberry
National Volcanic
Monument turned
10 years old in
June of 2001.

25 miles to Bend

A curious reminder of Mt. Newberry's eruption, the Lava Cast Forest rates near the top of our must–see local attractions. The volcanic tree molds are a rare and exotic sight, remnants of an ancient forest invaded by basalt lava flow. All levels of Mature Hikers will want to visit this fabulous site. Part of the trail is suitable for wheelchairs, but some sections might be too steep and narrow.

Geology
View
Trees

Getting there

- *Drive south from Bend about 15 miles on Hwy. 97 (3 miles south of Lava Lands Visitor Center).*
- *Take the Sunriver exit, turn left (east) and drive under 97 to connect to cinder Road 9720; drive 8.6 miles.*
- *Continue 0.7 miles on Road 9720–950 to a circle parking area.*

MILES
1

ELEV. GAIN
100 '

PERMIT
NW Forest Pass

OPEN
June to November/ December

MAPS
Map at trailhead, Deschutes National Forest Map.

The paved trail starts at the east end of the parking area in a lovely pine forest. Look for a box containing flyers with a map and an interpretive guide to the trail markers. The path, level in the beginning, snakes through the barren lava field where a few wildflowers and some currant bushes have adapted to a harsh existence. Scattered lodgepole and ponderosa pines also compete for limited moisture. The main attraction of the "forest," however, is the multitude of tree casts formed when flowing lava enveloped the live trees and quickly solidified into molds. The pines eventually burned, leaving a ghostly legacy in the lava casts.

At about the midpoint of the one–mile loop, stop at a viewpoint and look for Newberry's rim to the south and Mt. Bachelor and the Three Sisters to the northwest. Continue along a more challenging section of trail that contours over some small hills. Watch for horizontal tree molds here that formed around fallen pines. Notice, too, some venerable, gnarled ponderosa pines with their twisted "witch's broom" branches. The path arrives back at the parking area after one mile.

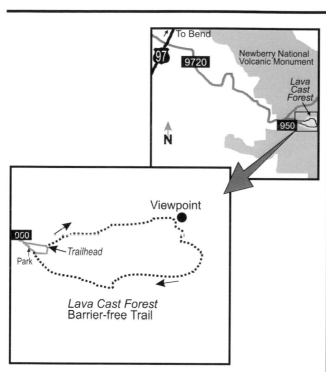

To Bend

97 9720

Newberry National
Volcanic Monument

Lava
Cast
Forest

N

950

Viewpoint

950

Trailhead

Park

Lava Cast Forest
Barrier-free Trail

Rock feature in Lava Cast Forest

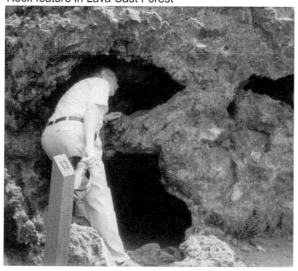

FACT FINDER

Rainforest Surprise

40 miles to Bend

Water

Forest

You can almost imagine yourself in a rainforest when you arrive at the headwaters of Jack Creek; at any rate, it's about as close as you'll come in dry Central Oregon. The mature trees and lush vegetation create a welcome oasis around the springs. All levels of Mature Hikers (from *Stroller* to *Adventure Hiker*) should make a point of visiting this magical site, a unique regional treasure.

Getting there

- *Drive west from Sisters on Highway 20 for 12.3 miles to a sign for Mt. Jefferson Wilderness Trailheads.*
- *Turn right (north) and follow Forest Road 12 for 4 miles.*
- *Turn left onto paved Road 1230; drive 0.6 miles.*
- *Turn left onto a red cinder road with a sign for Head of Jack Creek; drive 1.3 miles.*
- *Continue straight on Road 400 for about 0.4 miles to a cinder parking area.*

MILES
1

ELEV. GAIN
40'

PERMIT
NW Forest Pass

OPEN
June to November

MAPS
Deschutes National Forest Map,
USGS *Black Butte.*

Walk about one–fourth mile down to Jack Creek, then turn right and follow parallel to the stream on a smooth, needle–covered path. You'll enjoy the pleasant gurgle of flowing water as you pass among ponderosa pines, Douglas-firs and a few western larches, the only local conifer that loses its foliage in the fall. After walking through a natural "park" of granddaddy Doug-firs and ponderosa pines, step onto a quaint "Lincoln log" bridge that spans one branch of Jack Creek. Walk left on a short loop trail meandering between the headwaters and the convergence of the two forks flowing from them. You'll pass several giant western white pines (look for big cones) on your way to a small log bridge. The ferns and Pacific yews along the banks, the moss covered rocks and logs, the mist in the air, all combine to transport you out of arid Central Oregon. On a hot day, you might want to linger here.

The loop ends back at the first bridge. To see the actual springs of the headwaters, walk left along the creek for about 200 yards. Retrace your steps to return to the parking area.

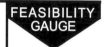
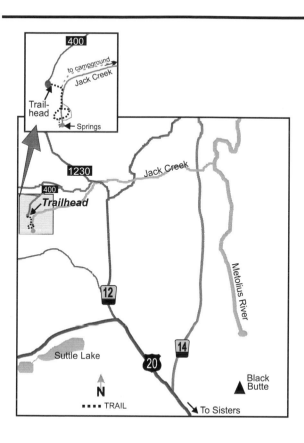

400

to campground

Jack Creek

Trail-
head

Springs

1230

Jack Creek

400

Trailhead

12

Metolius River

Suttle Lake

20

14

Black
Butte

N

▪▪▪▪ TRAIL

To Sisters

**TRAIL
CONDITION**
smooth dirt

**TRAILHEAD
FACILITIES**
*outhouse,
tables*

EXPOSURE
shaded

USE

moderate

STROLL

NOTES
*Mosquitoes likely
in mid-summer.*

Bridge over Jack Creek

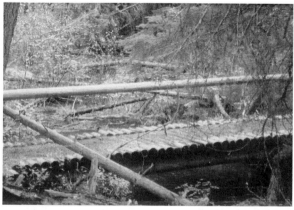

TIDBITS

The Douglas-fir was named by Scottish botanist, David Douglas. It is Oregon's state tree, and Oregon claims the national champion in both the coastal and Rocky Mountain Doug-fir categories. Not a true fir, it is the nation's most popular Christmas tree, and it furnishes more products used by humans than any other tree.

FACT FINDER

37 miles to Bend

Water Forest View

Getting there

- *Drive north from Bend on Highway 97 through Redmond to a sign for O'Neil (drive 16.3 miles from the junction of Hwy 20 and Hwy 97 near the Cascade Village Mall).*
- *Turn east (right) and drive 5 miles to Lone Pine Road.*
- *Turn north (left) and drive 8.6 miles.*
- *Turn north (left) on Hwy 26. Drive 4.6 miles and park at Rimrock Springs Wildlife Management Area on the right.*

MILES
1 – 1.5

ELEV. GAIN
100'

PERMIT
none

OPEN
all year

MAPS
Map on information board at trailhead, USGS *Gray Butte*.

If you crave solitude, you're likely to find it at this oasis in the desert. Bring binoculars and watch for deer and antelope plus waterfowl and numerous other birds, including eagles, owls, chickadees, goldfinches, white–faced ibis and black–headed grosbeak. The first one–half mile of trail is barrier–free with a crushed rock surface suitable for wheel chairs with pneumatic tires. You can stroll this path in winter when other trails are snowed–in; however, the surface could be snow–packed or muddy and the birds less evident.

The trail starts near the outhouse at the south end of the parking area. Walk east through a desert landscape of sagebrush and bunchgrass with sparse rabbit brush and a few juniper trees. The barrier–free trail ends after about one–half mile at a viewing platform. This is an ideal spot for bird watching with views of the ponds and marsh areas and the Ochoco Mountains beyond them to the east. Every *Stroller* should bring binoculars, and serious birders will want a camera with zoom lens. Those desiring a one–mile stroll will turn around at this platform.

For the 1.5 mile walk, continue to the right on a gravel/dirt path that passes through a gap in a fence and arrives within 0.25 mile at a second viewing platform. The ponds are clearly visible from here, as is Grizzly Mountain through the trees to the south. There is very little elevation change to this point, but the trail now winds up onto a juniper–covered bluff, turning west and then back to the north. The surface is smooth, but you should be prepared for mud in spring and winter. Once you crest the hill, you'll notice rock "frosting" on the ground and oddly shaped rock formations decorated with colorful moss and lichen. Take a faint side path to the left onto the rocks for views of Gray Butte, Broken Top, the Three Sisters and Mt. Jefferson. The trail gradually descends and rejoins the barrier–free trail a short distance to the east of the trailhead.

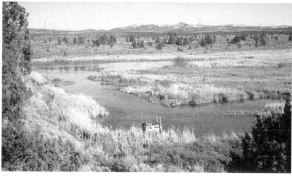

The pond at Rimrock Springs

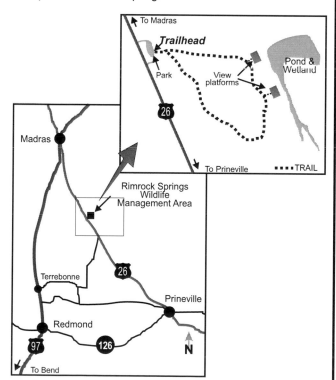

STROLL

FACT FINDER

10 miles to Bend

Geology View Forest

This outing provides a wonderful adventure in geology within a short drive from Bend. Relive a volcanic eruption as you trace the path of the lava flow. Imagine the astronauts here in the '60's practicing for the first moonwalk. Take in 360–degree views from the summit. *Strollers* can choose one or all of the walks. The Trail of the Molten Land has a side trail option that is somewhat steep; you will appreciate trekking poles here. Reserve some extra time to spend perusing exhibits in the Visitor Center. There are picnic tables under the pines in the car parking area.

Getting there

- *Drive 10 miles south of Bend on Hwy. 97.*
- *Turn right (west) into the Lava Lands Visitor Center. The toll booth attendant can sell you a NW Forest Pass if you don't have one. Follow the signs to the Visitor Center parking area.*
- *To drive up Lava Butte, turn right after passing the toll booth. During busy summer months, buses run regularly to the summit.*

MILES
1.5 total

ELEV. GAIN
175' total

PERMIT
NW Forest Pass

OPEN
mid–April to mid–October

MAPS
Deschutes National Forest Map,
USGS *Lava Butte.*

Trail of the Molten Land

You can access this paved trail on the west side of the Visitor Center. Just over the first rise, an expanse of lava stretches before you with views beyond of Mt. Bachelor, South Sister, Broken Top and the peaks of Middle and North Sister. As you stroll, enjoy the eerie effect of the jagged, contorted formations of "a–a" lava. Take time to read the interpretive signs along the trail and to identify the sparse vegetation — mostly pines, bitterbrush and currant. The trail winds through channels where the lava flowed when it spewed from a breach in the south side of Lava Butte. If you wish, take the side trail to the Phil Brogan viewpoint. You'll gain some elevation here, but you'll be rewarded with a closer look at the volcanic history as well as Cascade views and benches for resting. This detour adds 0.4 miles (included in the 1.5 mile total) to this one–half mile loop.

Trail of the Whispering Pines

As you finish the Trail of the Molten Land, follow the sign to the right for the one–third mile Trail of the Whispering Pines (or step out the back entrance of the Visitor Center). This paved, flat trail skirts the lava flow as it meanders through a ponderosa pine plantation planted in 1952. You'll notice just a few lodgepole pines amongst the ponderosas. The vegetation includes snowbrush, currant, manzanita and bitterbrush. There are educational markers and benches along this shady path, which crosses the Huntington Trail, a wagon and cattle road constructed in 1867.

Crater Rim Trail

Drive to the top of Lava Butte to stroll this one–fourth mile interpretive trail. You'll walk on red and black cinders plus a short, steep paved section with handrails accessing the lookout tower. The path loops around the steep crater of Lava Butte and affords terrific mountain views from pointy Mt. Thielsen in the south to Mt. Hood to the north.

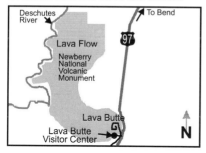

Trail of the Molten Lands

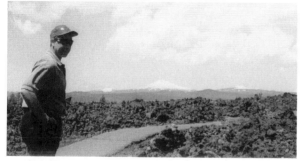

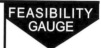

FEASIBILITY GAUGE

TRAIL CONDITION
paved or cinder

TRAILHEAD FACILITIES
restrooms, tables, exhibits

EXPOSURE
part shaded, part open

USE

heavy

Whispering Pines

NOTES
Trekking poles helpful for short steeper sections.

STROLL

Visitor Center Hours
Late April – late Sept.
Daily: 9am - 5pm
Call 541/593-2421
to verify opening date
and daily hours.

TIDBITS

Lava Butte, with its 180–foot deep crater, is an extinct cinder cone along a fissure from Newberry. The Lava Butte flow, a dramatic sight from the summit, is 30 – 100 feet deep and covers nine square miles.

FACT FINDER

IN
Bend

Water
Trees
View

This stroll meanders upstream along the Deschutes River as it passes through Drake Park near downtown Bend. You'll follow the river through a neighborhood then walk through Columbia Park and cross on a quaint footbridge. The mature trees in the parks and the ever–present waterfowl complement the enchanting Deschutes, Bend's pride and joy.

Getting there

- *Drive west on Franklin Avenue to downtown Bend.*
- *Just beyond Wall Street, turn north (right) into the Mirror Pond parking area.*

MILES
1.5

ELEV. GAIN
< 30'

PERMIT
none

OPEN
all year

MAPS
Bend City Map,
USGS ***Bend.***

Walk toward the river. Look for a bench and a view of North Sister, then go down a slope to the left and follow a paver path along the riverbank. Bend's first schoolhouse was built near here in the late 1800's; the log structure was also used by the *Bulletin* and Boy Scout groups before being abandoned in 1910. Take time to observe the stately homes on the far shore across Mirror Pond. On the park side, you'll pass a restroom and a performing arts platform before coming to a footbridge. Don't cross here; instead continue into the grass along the river's edge. When you reach the park boundary, turn right on the sidewalk and cross over the river. At Harmon Boulevard, carefully cross Galveston Avenue and walk south on Harmon to its intersection with Columbia. If you prefer to walk on a sidewalk, you can cross to the west side of the street here. Continue on to Columbia Park on the left. Stroll across the park toward a play area, keeping an eye out for flying frisbees, and walk down to the footbridge over the Deschutes. Note the boxy boulders of volcanic tuff on the west bank before walking through a short alley and turning left on Riverfront. This historic neighborhood of quaint houses was home to many of the mill workers in the mid–twentieth century.

Carefully cross Galveston Avenue and walk back into Drake Park. This time, if you wish, stay on the sidewalk and observe the regal ponderosa pines, western larches, Englemann spruces and western junipers, many of which are centenarians. The sidewalk will take you back to the Mirror Pond parking area.

"Big wheels" from early logging days

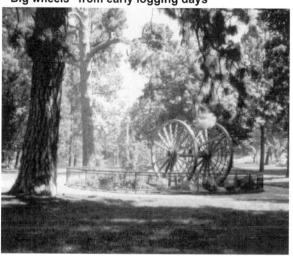

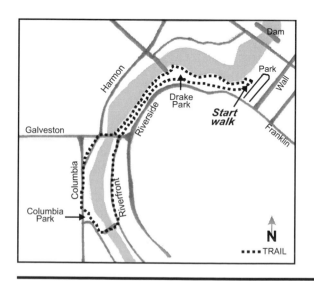

50 miles to Bend

Water
Forest
Geology

This lovely walk loops past two incredible waterfalls, one spilling into a secluded pool with no visible outlet. Lush vegetation, dense forest and sounds of water make it a good outing for a hot summer day. The walk is short, but it includes a few steeper, rocky sections. *Strollers* who may be unsteady on their feet should take a trekking pole or a companion for extra support.

Getting there

■ *Drive west from Sisters on Highway 242 to McKenzie Pass.*
■ *Continue down the other side about 13.5 miles to an often–crowded parking area on the right side of the highway (this is just past milepost 65).*
■ *Walk to the trailhead across the road.*

MILES
1.2

ELEV. GAIN
200'

PERMIT
NW Forest Pass

OPEN
June/July to October

MAPS
Geo Graphics *Three Sisters Wilderness Map*, *Willamette National Forest Map*, USGS *Linton Lake*.

Walk counter–clockwise on the path from the roadside trailhead. As you move up onto a lava flow known as Deadhorse Grade, watch for vine maple and Oregon grape plus a variety of leafy foliage not seen on the east side of the mountains. Take a side trail to an overlook of Lower Proxy Falls. If you're feeling adventurous, you can scramble down a small trail to water level. Near the water, yew trees join the predominately fir forest.

Continue on the main trail to Upper Proxy Falls, which, like Lower Proxy, drops about two hundred feet over a cliff into a tree–darkened pool. You'll wonder why the pool never overfills with such a large amount of water flowing in. Evidently, water seeps through the porous lava and resurfaces in some springs down the canyon. When you can pull yourself away from this magical spot, walk back to the main trail and continue on to the trailhead. Rhododendron, bear grass and vanilla leaf bloom along here in early summer.

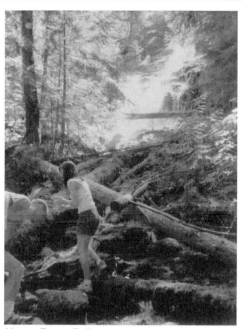

Upper Proxy Falls

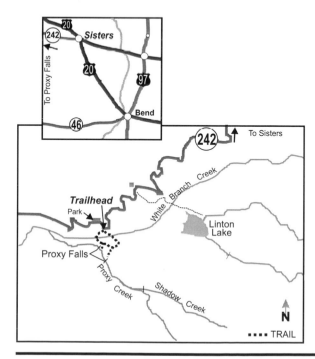

To Sisters

Sisters

To Proxy Falls

Bend

Trailhead
Park

Linton
Lake

Proxy Falls

Proxy Creek

White Branch Creek

Shadow Creek

N

•••• TRAIL

TRAIL CONDITION
some roots & rocks

TRAILHEAD FACILITIES
outhouse

EXPOSURE
shaded

USE
heavy

STROLL

NOTES
Trekking poles helpful for some strollers; mosquitoes likely in mid-summer.

TIDBITS
Pacific yew trees grow west of the Cascade crest and you'll see them on just 3 outings in this guide. The *taxus brevifolia* is the only conifer to have "berries" for its fruit, and these bright red "arils" are treats for birds but highly toxic to humans. Yews of-ten grow near water under the shade of larger firs and hemlocks. The tough yew wood is used for bows, paddles and fence posts.

FACT FINDER

27 miles to Bend

Water Forest

This outing opens the joys of the wilderness to *Walkers* and most *Strollers* as you follow along boisterous Fall Creek to several scenic falls. There's a gradual uphill slope near the beginning of the trail. Those who walk to the additional falls will have to gain some more elevation. The Green Lakes Trail is hugely popular, so it's best to take this outing in the late fall or at least on a mid–week day instead of during the weekend.

Getting there

- *Drive west from Bend on Highway 46/Century Drive, driving 4.5 miles past Mt Bachelor Ski Resort.*
- *Turn right into the Green Lakes Trailhead parking area. Find the Green Lakes trail, which starts on the left (west) side of the parking area. Fill out the free Three Sisters Wilderness permit.*

MILES
1 +

ELEV. GAIN
75' +

PERMIT
NW Forest Pass

OPEN
July to October/ November

MAPS
Geo Graphics *Three Sisters Wilderness Map,*
Deschutes National Forest Map,
USGS *Broken Top.*

Cross Fall Creek on a log bridge, then walk up a gradual slope for 100 or so yards. The trail flattens out and follows above the creek through a forest of lodgepole pines, mountain hemlocks and subalpine firs. The relatively smooth path leaves the creek for a short distance; when you come to the creek again, turn right and walk down to a viewpoint above the falls. Rocks form a natural staircase down to a lower viewpoint. Some folks will not want to attempt this without assistance from a friend or trekking poles. At this lower level you'll feel the spray as the water tumbles over a 45–foot, moss–encrusted rock bluff. Take a minute to enjoy the negative ions produced by the turbulent water. At the upper viewing area, notice the unique five–forked hemlock tree. This is a possible picnic site if you don't mind sitting on the ground.

To see two additional falls, continue up the trail through several switchbacks, past some noisy cascades, to a viewpoint above a short, broad waterfall that's about 15 feet high. You'll notice that the forest here is almost exclusively hemlock with a few small firs in the understory. Walk another 100 or so yards to a lovely 20–foot falls. This is a good turnaround point for the outing unless the adventurer in you wants to explore farther along rushing Fall Creek .

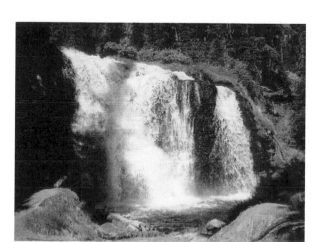

First waterfall on Fall Creek

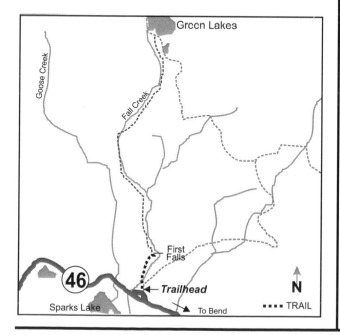

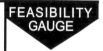
TRAIL CONDITION
mostly smooth, some roots & rocks

TRAILHEAD FACILITIES
outhouse

EXPOSURE
shaded

USE
heavy

STROLL

NOTES
Trekking pole helpful; mosquitoes likely in mid-summer.

TIDBITS

The Wilderness Act of 1964 defines wilderness as "an area where the earth and its community of life are untrammeled by man...." Man loves and uses the Three Sisters Wilderness, with its 260 miles of trails, 4 major peaks and Oregon's largest glacier, more than any other in the region.

61

19 | SOUTH TWIN LAKE

39 miles to Bend

Forest Water

This pristine lake is a perfect blue circle of water filling one of two petite volcanic craters just north of large Wickiup Reservoir. The short stroll around the lake will leave you enough time to visit Billy Quinn's grave site at Osprey Point (see Tidbit), and enjoy lunch in the quaint lakeside restaurant at Twin Lakes Resort near the start of the trail.

Getting there

- *Drive south from Bend on Highway 97 about 17 miles.*
- *Turn right on Vandevert Road (#42) and drive 1 mile.*
- *Turn left on South Century Drive (which curves to the right within 1 mile) and drive 20 miles.*
- *Turn left at sign for Twin Lakes and drive about 2 miles; park at Twin Lakes Resort or South Twin Campground.*

MILES
1

ELEV. GAIN
20'

PERMIT
NW Forest Pass

OPEN
June to Oct/Nov

MAPS
Deschutes National Forest Map, USGS *Davis Mountain.*

The trail begins on the water side of the resort and campground. Walk to the south to go counter clock-wise around the lake. A sandy path follows above the sloped beach past rental cabins in the trees. Foliage growing on the shore includes bitterbrush, manzanita, wild roses and snowbrush. On the west shore you can walk near the water, but you'll have to step over some downed logs. We recommend staying on the official path for flat and easy walking.

When the path takes you into the trees, watch for ponderosa and lodgepole pines as well as Douglas–firs and a few alders. The view back across the lake includes Cultus Mountain to the west. Just beyond the midpoint of the trek, there's a bench for resting near the water's edge.

Stay in the woods until you come even with the day use picnic area, then move down to the beach. On warm summer days, swimmers, boaters and sun seekers hang out here. It's usually a tame crowd. The lake's rainbow trout population makes it popular with fishermen. Motor boats, however, are not allowed. A sign points to North Twin Lake (which affords an optional trek, adding about 1 mile). Continue skirting the beach, walking between the campground and the water, to return to your starting point.

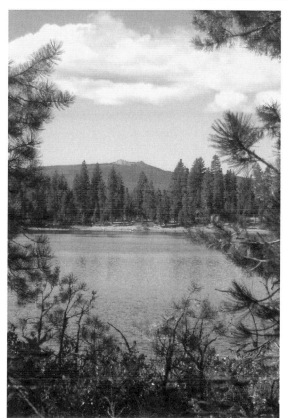

South Twin Lake

FEASIBILITY GAUGE

TRAIL CONDITION
mostly smooth dirt

TRAILHEAD FACILITIES
outhouse, campground, store, restaurant

EXPOSURE
open and airy forest

USE
light

STROLL

NOTES
Trekking poles nice for side slope. Mosquitoes likely in summer.

TIDBITS

Billy Quinn was a young sheep-herder who was accidentally shot while hunting in the Crane Prairie area in 1894. For an interesting side trip to the site of his grave, continue west on 42, turn north on 46 and right at Osprey Point. The short stroll to the grave con-tinues to the headwaters of the Quinn River.

To **42**

South Twin Lake

Trailhead

Resort

Detail

To Bend

Deschutes River

97

46

Crane Prairie Reservoir

Osprey Point
(Billy Quinn Grave)

42

Vandevert Road

South Twin Lake

42

43

Wickiup Reservoir

N

■ ■ ■ TRAIL

29 miles to Bend

Forest Water

This short–and–sweet outing is definitely off the beaten path. The lovely, lazy Fall River, though popular with anglers, is too shallow for boating and other recreation, so you'll most likely enjoy strolling in peaceful solitude. On a hot day, this clear and cold spring–fed stream may tempt you to linger on the bank or even wade in the refreshing water.

Getting there

- *Drive south from Bend on Highway 97 about 17.5 miles.*
- *Turn right on Vandevert Road (Rd. 42) and drive 1 mile.*
- *Turn left on South Century Drive (which curves to the right within 1 mile) and drive 10.8 miles.*
- *Turn left into Fall River Campground (just before milepost 16). Parking area is straight ahead.*

**MILES
*1.2***

**ELEV. GAIN
*20'***

**PERMIT
*none***

**OPEN
*April to
Nov/Dec***

MAPS
Deschutes National Forest Map, USGS ***Pistol Butte.***

The trail begins to the southwest side of the parking area opposite an outhouse. It's rather indistinct, but you can walk down to the river and intersect it. A bridge crosses to a path on the far bank, but for this outing stay on the north side. Since Fall River doesn't lose much elevation in this stretch, it's much calmer and quieter than most Central Oregon Rivers. Noisy rapids won't distract you from other sounds of nature, but you will notice the burble of several springs that feed this stream. Follow along the river until the trail peters out, then move onto the upper trail to the north. Look for an osprey nest high up in a dead tree, and note the magnificent old–growth ponderosa pines that rule over the airy forest.

When you reach the historic guard station, explore the grounds, then walk to the southwest corner to "discover" the headwaters. From this point, Fall River flows just twelve miles to its mouth in the Deschutes River. Brown, brook and rainbow trout fill its waters and tempt anglers.

Walk back to your car the way you came. Then, for an extra treat, visit the Fall River Fish Hatchery (go back east on Road 42 to the sign). Several kinds of trout are raised here for stocking mountain lakes. Purchase a handful of fish food to create an entertaining feeding frenzy in the tanks.

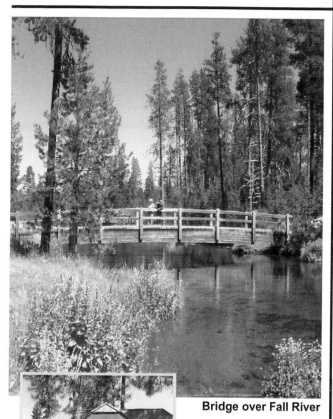

Bridge over Fall River

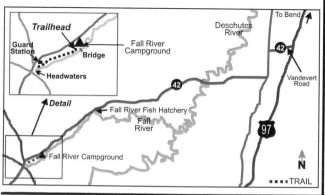

Fall River Guard Station

TRAIL
CONDITION
*mostly
smooth dirt*

TRAILHEAD
FACILITIES
*outhouse,
campground*

EXPOSURE
airy forest

USE
𝕏
light

STROLL

NOTES
*Mosquitoes likely
i n   s u m m e r
months.*

TIDBITS

The Fall River Guard Station was built by CCC crews in the 1930's at the picturesque headwaters. It served as a base for fire fighting and other forest administration. The Forest Service has recently renovated this historic structure which can be rented by private citizens.

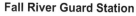

Trailhead
Guard
Station
Bridge
Headwaters
Fall River
Campground
Deschutes
River
To Bend
42
Vandevert
Road
Detail
Fall River Fish Hatchery
Fall
River
42

Fall River Campground
N
····TRAIL

FACT FINDER

IN
Bend

Water
Trees

It's amazing that within the city limits of a town known for its outdoor enthusiasts, it's still possible to enjoy wild beauty without encountering many people. But that's often the case on this boisterous section of the Deschutes – we almost hate to share the secret. If you're running errands on the south side of Bend, take a refreshing break and walk this scenic trail.

Getting there

- *From the traffic circle above the Old Mill District (Bond Street/Reed Market Road/Brookswood Blvd.), take Brookswood to the south.*
- *Drive 2.5 miles and turn west (right) on Sweetbriar.*
- *Turn left on Snowbrush; turn right on Pine Drive and park to the right (limited parking; don't block drives).*

MILES
1–2

ELEV. GAIN
30'

PERMIT
none

OPEN
all year

MAPS
Bend City Map,
USGS ***Bend.***

Locate the gravel/dirt road heading north off Pine. Go around a gate and walk down about 50 yards to a hairpin curve then another 50 yards to where the path levels and follows the river to the north. Here you'll notice the diversion channels where Central Oregon Irrigation District diverts water to its canal system. There is also a fish screen – not accessible to the public – which directs fish back into the river.

The first time we attempted to walk this trail, we were turned back by emergency crews conducting a rescue on the river. All too frequently, rafters put in upstream at Meadow Camp planning to float to Bend. Many are thrown from their craft in the rapids, and some become trapped against the grate of the canal intake. A safe stroll along the bank certainly beats fighting for your life in the raging whitewater.

The river becomes a bit calmer as you walk north through manzanita, snowbrush, bitterbrush and currant. Pines and aspens have been planted to screen the large aqueduct to the right. Across the river you'll notice dramatic cliffs and large ponderosa pines. A few homes are visible above the cliffs.

Near the one-half mile mark, walk out onto a

small viewing platform and enjoy the river sights and sounds. You can turn around here for a one mile stroll or continue until you see the footbridge over the river down to the left. This point marks the turn–around for a two–mile walk. (To get to the bridge – see *Outing 33* – you must walk another ¼ mile and connect to a path leading down to the river.) As you retrace your steps to the trailhead, look across the river just north of the viewing pier to spot an osprey nest at the top of a dead pine tree.

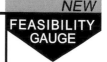
FEASIBILITY GAUGE

TRAIL CONDITION
smooth dirt

TRAILHEAD FACILITIES
none

EXPOSURE
open

USE
🚶🚲
light

STROLL

NOTES
Watch for mud in winter and spring. You may appreciate trekking poles for a short slope at trails' beginning.

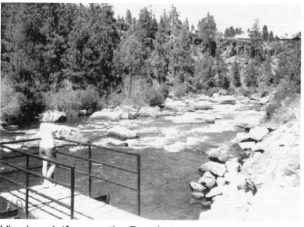

Viewing platform on the Deschutes

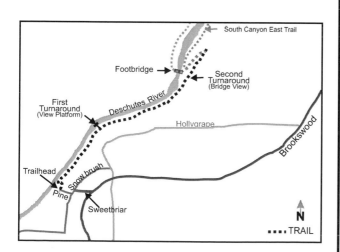

TIDBITS

At Meadow Camp, the Deschutes is deceptively calm. A sign warns, "Dangerous Falls Ahead." Class 4 & 5 rapids make the 4 mile stretch of river between here and the Old Mill District suitable only for experienced kayakers. Rafts and inner tubes are prohibited.

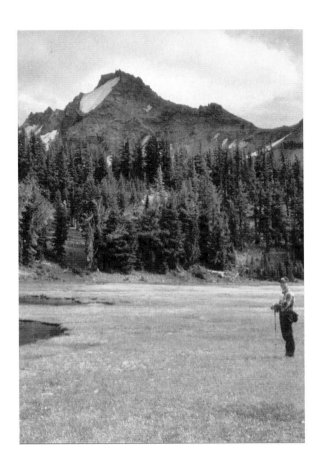

If strolls are appetizers, then walks must be the pasta course — very tasty and satisfying yet leaving room for more. We think you'll love these outings for their variety and scenic beauty. From a desert trek to a view climb to several river rambles, the walks will undoubtedly raise your spirits as well as your pulse rate. Many folks would be thrilled to have such a pleasant way to exercise so close to home or hotel. Take these fourteen walks and we can almost guarantee you'll be addicted. Don't fret; the meat course is next with eighteen choices. In addition, the strolls will give you some tempting dessert options.

WALKS

Part Three

FACT FINDER

IN
Bend

This short, easy walk provides an opportunity to experience river life within the city limits. The path wends along between the tall rock cliffs of Awbrey Butte and the Deschutes River, with its large population of water fowl. The rapids near the trail's beginning make an ideal playground for folks practicing kayak maneuvers. Winter is a good time to walk here, although the trail can be muddy.

Water Geology

Getting there

- *From the intersection of Business 97 (NE 3rd Street) and NE Greenwood Avenue, drive west 0.6 mile.*
- *Turn right on Wall Street and drive north 0.3 mile to NW Portland Avenue.*
- *Turn left and drive west over the river 0.2 mile to NW First Street. Turn right and drive north 0.3 miles to a small cul-de-sac parking area at First Street Rapids.*

MILES
1.7

ELEV. GAIN
40'

PERMIT
none

OPEN
all year

MAPS
Bend City Map,
USGS *Bend.*

Walk to the left down a gradual incline to reach the smooth woodchip trail. Turn left and follow the river through a typical Central Oregon landscape of western juniper trees, rabbit brush and bitterbrush. Soon, rugged rock cliffs emerge on the left, then tall rock banks become visible across the river. When the river makes a slight bend, look at the far cliff top to see townhomes which replaced a vintage log home). A postcard scene unfolds below this landmark — tall ponderosa pines against the basalt cliff giving way to a still, rock–dotted river pool, an area of high quality urban wildlife habitat for otter, osprey, owl and marmot.

When the river turns to the east, look toward the far bend at "Swan Pond," created by the North Canal Dam and named for the four trumpeter swans that frequent the pool. The trail continues left up a fairly steep bank above a golf course. You can turn around here or continue up the hill 0.2 miles to Mt. Washington Drive and turn there. This higher path affords a nice view of a golf fairway. Take care coming down; the woodchips can be a bit slippery on the steeper terrain. When you arrive back at the trailhead, stay to the left and walk fifty feet or so on a gravel path to an overlook of the rapids. Steidl Dam is visible just to the south.

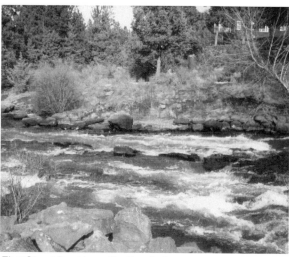

First Street Rapids on the Deschutes

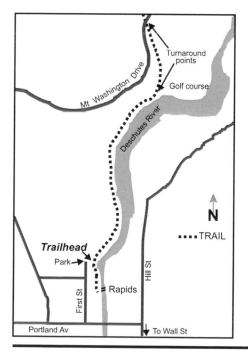

FACT FINDER

28 miles to Bend

Geology
Water
View
Forest

Every Mature Hiker should make this intriguing outing a priority. *Walkers* and many *Strollers* will appreciate having a "mountain" adventure on a relatively easy trail. Experiencing the unique geology around Sparks Lake is sufficient reward even without the stunning lake and snow cap views. After the outing, you'll know why this Cascade lake was a favorite spot for Oregon's former photographer laureate, Ray Atkeson. (*Bonus*: look for the most elegant outhouse in the forest at this trailhead.)

Getting there

- *Drive west from Bend 28 miles on Highway 46/Century Drive (go about 4 miles past Mt Bachelor Ski Resort).*
- *Turn left on Road 400 to Sparks Lake. Stay left for just over 1 mile to a trailhead parking area near the boat landing.*
- *Locate the trailhead at the west end of the parking area.*

MILES
1.2–2.3

ELEV. GAIN
50'

PERMIT
NW Forest Pass

OPEN
July to October/ November

MAPS
Geo Graphics *Three Sisters Wilderness Map*, Deschutes National Forest Map, USGS *Broken Top*.

Stay to the right on the paved trail and walk one–fourth mile to an overlook with benches and views of South Sister and Broken Top. Lodgepole pine trees keep company here with rugged canyons and crevices formed by glacier movement and lava flow from erupting Cascade volcanoes. The pavement ends about fifty yards beyond the viewpoint as the trail continues through pines, subalpine firs and mountain hemlocks. You'll be fascinated by the unique formations, caves, cracks and gullies in the lava flow. Look for the deeper canyon near Sparks Lake where water flows in good snow years. As you come to an inlet of the lake, watch for a small rock bridge over a crack perpendicular to the main canyon. In good snow years, Sparks Lake is a blue gem with a snowcap backdrop. It has an eerie beauty in low–snow years, when algae makes a multicolored film on its muddy bottom, which may be visible on this shallow south finger.

At a sign for Davis Canyon, turn left to follow this scenic spur trail through an incredible fifteen–foot canyon. You'll feel you are miles from civilization in this cool wonderland that supports some leafy shrubs and a few subalpine firs. When you leave the canyon, stay to the right to walk a 1.1 mile loop (or keep left to get back to the trailhead in 0.5 mile). You'll pass a dramatic boulder pit and crest a rock bluff before returning to the main loop. Proceed to the right through rugged rock walls and pressure ridges to return to the trailhead.

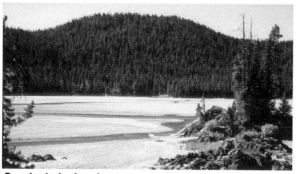

Sparks Lake in a low-snow year

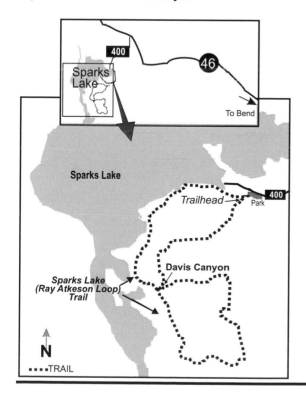

TRAIL CONDITION
mostly smooth, some roots & rocks

TRAILHEAD FACILITIES
outhouse

EXPOSURE
airy forest

USE
moderate

NOTES
Mosquitoes likely in mid-summer.

WALK

TIDBITS

Sparks Lake received its name from local pioneer E.H. Sparks, who was known as "Lige." Sparks was a cattleman and early owner of Swamp Ranch, now Black Butte Ranch. At one time, Sparks as-sociate A.S. Holmes grazed cattle in the meadows around Sparks Lake.

Quick Canyon Getaway

FACT
FINDER

6 miles to Bend

Water
Forest
Geology

Just two miles outside Bend's city limits, Tumalo State Park is a locals' favorite for swimming and picnicking. Fine summer weather can bring crowds to the day–use area, but few of the frolickers venture onto the one–mile river trail. Following the Deschutes through this secluded canyon makes for a pleasant outing any time of year. Day passes can be purchased for three dollars at a fee station near the entrance.

Getting there

- *Turn northwest on O.B. Riley Road at its intersection with Business 97 (across from Bend River Promenade).*
- *Drive 3.9 miles to Tumalo State Park.*
- *Turn left into the day–use area and park toward the south (far) end of the parking lot.*

MILES
1.8

ELEV. GAIN
< 50'

PERMIT
state park pass

OPEN
all year

MAPS
Deschutes National Forest Map,
USGS *Tumalo.*

Walk from the parking lot toward the river and turn left (south) on a path that parallels the Deschutes. On a warm summer day, the sounds of merriment will lead you to a popular swimming hole with a broad grassy bank. Look for the dirt river trail at the far end of the grass and proceed upstream.

After a short distance the path brings you to a private driveway. Follow the pavement to a bridge then veer left, staying on the east side of the river. Large ponderosa pines and western junipers keep company with currant, Oregon grape and red osier dogwood in this quiet corridor. The river bank slopes up to rim rock on the left. A small butte on the far side gives way to canyon walls as you continue upriver. The trail stays fairly level, although the water moves along at a good pace, churning to foamy rapids in places. A wood bench along the way makes a nice resting/viewing spot. A second bench marks a good turnaround point, although the adventurous can scramble up tumbled basalt boulders for a better view of the river. Be sure to look for stable hand and foot holds if you climb through the rocks!

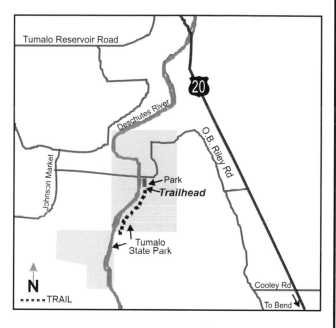

Tumalo Reservoir Road

Deschutes River

Johnson Market

O.B. Riley Rd

20

Park

Trailhead

Tumalo
State Park

Cooley Rd

To Bend

N

----- TRAIL

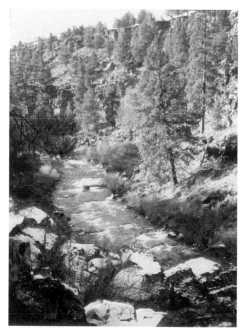

Deschutes River canyon at Tumalo State Park

IN
Bend

When folks think of Bend and the qualities that define our city, the mighty Deschutes River often looms large in their thoughts. In its variously boisterous and serene journey through our region, the beloved river supports numerous species of fish and wildlife and provides multiple recreation opportunities. This rejuvenating walk along its banks transports you to another place, refreshing your spirit in the process. If the river captures your imagination and affection, you'll want to consider *Outings 4, 7, 16, 22, 24, 26, 27, 29 and 50.*

Water
Geology
Trees

Getting there

- *From the intersection of Highway 97 and SW Colorado Avenue, drive west on Colorado 1.7 miles.*
- *At the circle intersection of Century Drive and Colorado, drive south (left) on Century 0.3 mile to 2nd circle.*
- *Go around circle and turn onto Reed Market Road; go right on Mt. Bachelor and drive 0.4 mile; turn left into the conference center parking area. If this is full, check with Guest Registration across the street for available parking (or go back to first circle - Reed & Mt. Bachelor - and park in a parallel space along Mt. Bachelor; walk toward the river to locate the trail).*

MILES
2.2

ELEV. GAIN
100'

PERMIT
none

OPEN
all year

MAPS
Bend City Map,
USGS *Bend.*

Find the trail across the street from Guest Registration; walk north toward the Reed/Mt. Bachelor traffic circle, then take the sidewalk down to the river. Take a quick look to the left at the jointed columnar cliffs on the west bank. This rock, called tuff, resulted when dense ash flow settled and solidified. Pass through a gate on your right to access the path that parallels the Deschutes. Signs along the route provide descriptions of points of interest. Walking south, you'll pass a lodge and some homes, which fortunately don't diminish the peace and beauty of the river. A grassy bank with a picnic table makes a fine place to look for otters, herons, beavers and other wildlife that thrive here.

As you continue upstream through ponderosa and juniper trees, watch for a footbridge on the far side of the river. The bridge spans a channel of water re–entering the river after passing through a hydro power plant buried underground. The well–disguised plant provides electricity for about 2500 homes.

As the river loses elevation and becomes noisy, you'll have to gain some elevation. Walk up a bluff of basalt boulders and turn left on a dirt trail to visit an overlook of frothy rapids. When you rejoin the main path, look for manzanita, with its shiny, evergreen leaves, on the slope to the right. The trail continues to climb a bit, then curves back north into Mt. Bachelor Village. Look to the right over the roofs of the town homes for yellow pumice cliffs in the far canyon wall. Pumice formed when gas expanded in erupting magma, creating a bubbly rock that absorbed water as it reached the surface. Walk past tennis courts and a swimming pool back to your starting point.

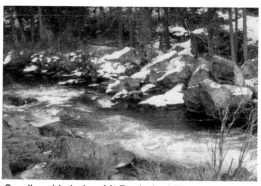

Small rapids below Mt Bachelor Village

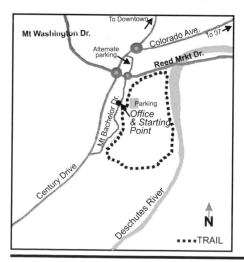

▪▪▪▪TRAIL

TRAIL
CONDITION
smooth

TRAILHEAD
FACILITIES
*table &
benches
along trail*

EXPOSURE
*mostly
shaded*

USE

*moderate
to heavy*

NOTES

Trail can be muddy or snow-packed in winter and spring.

TIDBITS

One of several kinds of volcanic rock along the river, tuff was quarried and used locally as a building stone in the early 1900's. Pumice rock is still mined in the region. The Deschutes National Forest is the largest supplier of pumice in the Pacific Northwest.

WALK

Canyon Overlook

IN
Bend

Outstanding returns are guaranteed when you invest an hour on the Sawyer river trail. Among your rewards are eye–level and bird's–eye views of the Deschutes and glimpses of volcanic cliffs and snow–clad mountains. The *Awbrey reach* section of the river is popular with fishermen and kayakers, as well as children who like to play on the weathered boulders lining the river in Sawyer Park. Passing calmly through the park, then churning noisily into canyon country, the river shows several of its many faces to users of this delightful trail.

Water
Geology
View

Getting there

- *At the Bend River Promenade Mall on Business 97 (between Butler Market Road and River Mall Drive), turn northwest on O.B. Riley Road.*
- *Drive 0.4 miles to Sawyer Park.*
- *Turn left (west) into the parking lot.*

MILES
about 3

ELEV. GAIN
<100'

PERMIT
none

OPEN
all year

MAPS
Bend City Map,
USGS *Bend.*

Cross the footbridge over the Deschutes River and walk straight ahead about fifty yards. A short distance to the east, an apple orchard was planted on the Collins and Stearns Ranch in 1900. Cut across the grassy playing field on your right to the Deschutes River Trail (there's a trail marker on the far side of the field). Turn right onto a smooth woodchip path that emerges from the trees into an open landscape of rabbit brush, bitterbrush, currant and sagebrush, with sparse ponderosa pines and junipers. After a short distance you'll find yourself walking on a broad shelf between a rugged rock wall and the river canyon. Look for leafy vegetation here, including a few wild roses. A short descent brings you to Archie Briggs Road and the Wyndemere neighborhood.

The trail continues across the street, leaving the river and winding through part of the subdivision. You'll soon come back to a broader, deeper canyon and views of Broken Top, the Three Sisters, Mt. Washington, Three Fingered Jack, Mt. Jefferson and Mt. Hood. The path slopes down into a gully, turns north, then climbs back up to parallel a cliff. Soon, the trail and the river make a 90–degree turn to the west. You will enjoy the mountain and river views from this vantage point. This is a good place to turn around, although the path continues along the route of a recently–buried irrigation canal.

As you return to Sawyer Park, resist the urge to rest a spell in one of Wyndemere's charming gardens. Maturity has its privileges, but trespassing isn't one of them.

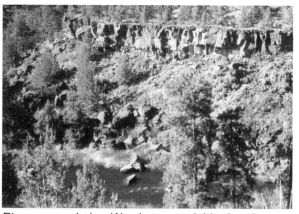

River canyon below Wyndemere neighborhood

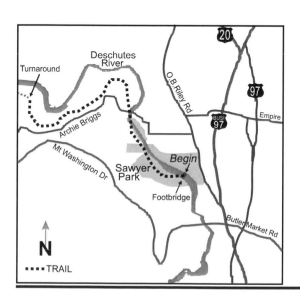

TRAIL CONDITION
smooth, woodchip

TRAILHEAD FACILITIES
outhouse, tables

EXPOSURE
open

USE
🚶 🚲
moderate to heavy

NOTES
Trail can be muddy or snow-packed in winter and spring; one street crossing.

TIDBITS

Sawyer Park is a 61–acre community park named for early *Bulletin* publisher Robert W. Sawyer. Wildlife finding favor with the riverside habitat include owls, deer, mink and humming-birds. Four diversions south of the park cause a dramatic fluctuation in flow through this river section.

WALK

Ancient People's Shelter

7 miles to Bend

Water Geology Forest

How many places can you drive just past the city limits and walk through a rugged setting perfect for a western movie set? Yes, there are houses visible here, but you won't want to miss the unusual natural scenery, including a shelter used by Native Americans. This trail is accessible for most of the year. All levels of Mature Hikers will enjoy a wonderful outing that doesn't include a long drive.

Getting there

- *Drive west from Bend on Highway 46/Century Drive (from the traffic circle where Century Drive and SW Colorado intersect, drive about 3.5 miles).*
- *Just before Widgi Creek Golf Course, turn left at the sign for Meadow Picnic Area. Follow this gravel road 1.2 miles to a parking area.*

MILES 2.2

ELEV. GAIN < 60'

PERMIT none

OPEN most of the year

MAPS
Deschutes National Forest Map, USGS **Benham Falls.**

Walk up a slope south of the parking area to follow the trail above the calm Deschutes. As you stroll through a forest of ponderosa pines with manzanita and bitterbrush, you'll soon notice a lava flow to the left that separates the river from an overflow channel. After passing a tumbled–boulder slope on the right, walk through red osier dogwoods and nightshade to cross a dammed pond located below the Seventh Mountain Resort. The trail continues around a rocky bluff and follows above the channel. The river is hidden by the lava flow here, but homes in the Deschutes River Woods subdivision can be seen high atop the far bank. Notice the thick stand of fir trees lower on the bank and the irrigation flume above them. This one–mile flume was built in 1905 and rebuilt in 1947.

The trail meanders along a rock bluff on the right, at one point passing under rock outcroppings, and eventually coming to an ancient rock shelter. The items excavated from this shelter are on display at the DesChutes Historical Museum in Bend. The path switchbacks up onto a bluff where there are interpretive signs and a rustic bench. Though hidden by the lava island, the falls can be heard from this overlook. For a glimpse of the rapids, you'll have to carefully pick your way through rocks and brush toward the sound of water. The parking area beyond the falls is the turnaround point for this outing. If you walk in autumn, you'll enjoy a large stand of aspen trees upriver, resplendent in their golden fall finery. As you return downriver, watch for several contorted ponderosas, quirky caricatures of their straight–laced cousins. The tangled branches, called witch's broom, result from mistletoe infestation.

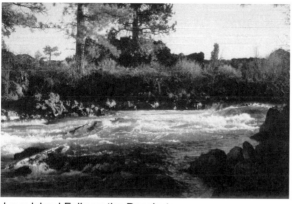

Lava Island Falls on the Deschutes

FEASIBILITY GAUGE

TRAIL CONDITION
mostly smooth, some rocks

TRAILHEAD FACILITIES
outhouse

EXPOSURE
mostly shaded

USE
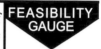
moderate to heavy

NOTES
Trail can be muddy or snow-packed in winter and spring.

TIDBITS

The *Riviere des Chutes*, as French Canadian traders called the Deschutes, flows from its source in Little Lava Lake 240 miles to the Columbia River. Fed by 1000 springs, it maintains a consistent flow due to porous lava that absorbs high flow. Nearly all of its feeder streams except the Crooked River originate in the Cascades.

WALK

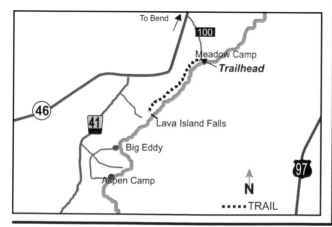

To Bend

100

Meadow Camp
Trailhead

46

41

Lava Island Falls

Big Eddy

97

Aspen Camp

N

•••••TRAIL

State Park in the City

IN
Bend

View
Geology

Walking up Pilot Butte is a local tradition for Bendites, so much so that if there were a Fraternal Order of Butte Walkers, it would have thousands of members. This means you're unlikely to have the trail to yourself; just think of it as a social hike. The challenge with this outing is, of course, the elevation gain. Sunscreen is imperative, and it's probably best to avoid the midday heat of summer. Casual *Walkers* will want to take it slowly; it's a good idea to work up to this trek by taking several of the easier walks in the guide first. You'll be rewarded not only with great views but with a feeling of exhilaration and accomplishment as well.

Getting there

- *Drive east through Bend on Greenwood Avenue/ Highway 20 past Pilot Butte.*
- *Turn north (left) on NE Azure, then left on NE Savannah and left on NE Linnea.*
- *Park in a paved lot with trailhead at the southwest end. When leaving, turn right on Arnette to go back to town.*

MILES
2

ELEV. GAIN
500'

PERMIT
none

OPEN
all year

MAPS
Bend City Map,
USGS *Bend.*

Walk one–eighth mile on a paved path to a fork. We suggest taking the nature trail to the right. It's smooth dirt and has several shaded sections. You might want to pick up the self–guided trail guide and read about the numbered points of interest. Plan to climb steadily except for one 100' flat section (this will give you something to look forward to). If you're not in top shape, you'll enjoy taking breaks at several of the five benches spread along the trail. The first bench overlooks a school playing field and provides views to the east of Pine Mountain, Powell Butte with its cultivated fields, and the Ochocos. From the second bench, look for Mt. Bachelor on your far left all the way around to Mt. Hood and Powell Butte to the right. The third bench faces Broken Top and looks down Greenwood Avenue toward Bend city center. The fourth bench looks south down Fifteenth Street with a view of Lava Butte, and the fifth affords views of Bessie Butte, Kelsey Butte and the Paulina Mountains.

The sparse trees on Pilot Butte are western junipers

and ponderosa pines. The high desert "brush trio" is prevalent here: sagebrush, bitterbrush and rabbit brush. Also look for red currant, fescue, bluebunch wheat-grass, penstemon, sand lily, yarrow and paintbrush.

Take time to enjoy views at the summit, where a marker dedicates the park to Bend pioneer, Terrence Foley. Map lovers will enjoy identifying buttes and mountains on the Deschutes National Forest Map. It's also fun to pick out various landmarks around town. If you want to take a different route down, start out on the dirt path alongside the paved road. When

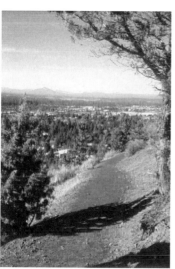

you come to a behemoth concrete water tank with hook–shaped vents on top, turn left onto the paved footpath and follow it back to the parking lot.

Trail on west side of Pilot Butte

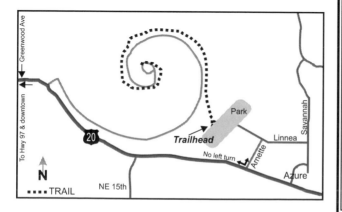

TRAIL CONDITION
smooth

TRAILHEAD FACILITIES
porta–potty

EXPOSURE
mostly open

USE
heavy

NOTES
Trekking poles helpful for walking down; in winter when there's snow on the north side, take paved path to the left.

TIDBITS

Called Red Butte in the early days, Bend's famous landmark became known as Pilot Butte by the turn of the century. For 3 brief years in the '60's, a ski jump was built and utilized on the northwest side; snow was trucked from the Tumalo Falls area. The butte is a recent basalt cone of red and black cinders.

WALK

FACT FINDER

The Spring-fed Cascade

10 miles
to
Bend

Water
Geology
Forest

Yes, you can drive to this site, but the walk along the river will give as much pleasure as seeing the falls. At times you'll feel like you're passing through unexplored territory. You might see a heron searching for dinner or a fisherman reeling in a trout. At the falls, there are several spots to sit on flat rocks and experience a sensory feast. Some folks will appreciate trekking poles for assistance on the log "staircase."

Getting there

- *Drive west from Bend on Highway 46/Century Drive (drive just over 5 miles from the traffic circle at the intersection of Century Drive and SW Colorado).*
- *Turn left on paved Road 41.*
- *Drive 1.6 miles and turn left on gravel Road 700.*
- *Follow the signs for Aspen Camp and drive about 0.8 miles to a parking area with outhouse. You may park at this upper area and follow a pumice path down to the river or drive to the lower parking area and walk past the boat landing to the trail marker on the south side.*

MILES
2.6

ELEV. GAIN
<75'

PERMIT
NW Forest Pass

OPEN
*April –
December*

MAPS
*Deschutes Nat-
ional Forest
Map,* USGS
Benham Falls.

Follow close to the river, quite calm in this stretch, through chartreuse–leafed aspens that turn gold in fall. The conifers here are ponderosa pines and grand firs, and the understory includes manzanita, snowbrush, bitterbrush, wild roses and currant. At times a narrow meadow with a willow backdrop separates the path from the river. When a slightly larger meadow opens up to the left, look for a shallow cave in the bank on your right. The river begins to run a bit faster as you come even with the lava flow on the far shore. Notice two grand Douglas–fir trees and a dramatic mossy cliff on the right. Walk up a log "staircase" (take your time here), to the first view of Dillon Falls. Continue forward along rock outcroppings for more views of the falls, which are really a series of white water drops. At the uppermost drop, look to the far bank to see springs spouting from the lava to join the river on its gleeful journey to Bend.

A picnic area and outhouse are located a hundred or so feet to the south of the falls. On the trip back to your car, instead of going down the "stairs," you can choose to stay left on the bicycle trail for a slightly different view. Listen for bicyclers and step to the side to let them pass. This upper route affords a view of a peaceful meadow across the Deschutes; several interpretive signs will enhance your enjoyment. You'll rejoin the lower path for the trek back to the parking area.

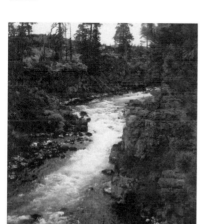

Dillon Falls on the Deschutes

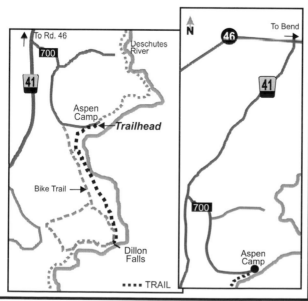

The Caldera Rim

FACT FINDER

38 miles to Bend

Water
Forest
Geology
View

This unique, short outing will tickle all your senses. As the trail traces the caldera rim of collapsed volcano Mt. Newberry, you'll enjoy almost continuous views of Paulina Lake and Paulina Peak, and you'll pass an unusual obsidian flow. *Hikers* will crest a cinder bluff to take in views of the distant southern Cascades. *Walkers* can wade on a pebbly beach or picnic in a meadow at the midpoint of their trek.

Getting there

- *Drive south from Bend 22 miles on Highway 97 to a sign for "Newberry Caldera."*
- *Drive east 12.5 miles on Road 21.*
- *At the entrance booth, purchase a NW Forest Pass if you don't already have one. Continue driving to the Little Crater Campground, about 1.5 miles, and turn left.*
- *Drive to the end of the campground and park in a graveled area at the trailhead.*

MILES
2.4 – 3.0

ELEV. GAIN
0 – 100'

PERMIT
NW Forest Pass

OPEN
June to November/December

MAPS
Deschutes National Forest Map,
USGS *East Lake.*

The rocky trail hugs the shoreline of turquoise Paulina Lake and skirts around a mixed forest of ponderosa, lodgepole and whitebark pines, as well as mountain hemlocks and subalpine firs. The path remains quite level, but you'll need to watch your step for rocks and roots. You'll walk past varied rock outcroppings for nearly three–quarters mile before coming to the Inter Lake Obsidian Flow, reaching from the Paulina shore eastward to East Lake. This is one of a very few places in the country where you actually walk on bits of shiny black obsidian glass. It won't hurt your shoes, but you don't want to fall on bare knees or hands. When the trail comes to a stretch of grassy beach, you might notice an unusual odor. This emanates from submarine warm springs; algae thrives along the shore here. Look to the right for a sheltered meadow, the undeveloped Warm Springs campground. *Walkers* can stop to picnic here or stroll a bit farther along the shore to a pebbly beach to wade or swim.

To continue the hike, keep to the trail that is back from shore a ways. The path becomes quite smooth here, and you'll start climbing as you enter the woods. When you come to a level stretch on the cinder bluff, stop to enjoy the views. Paulina Peak forms the backdrop across the lake to the left. A low place in the caldera rim provides views of Mt. McLoughlin, on the far left, and Mt. Thielsen, far right. This marks the turnaround point for the outing. If you do want to continue, you can wind down to North Cove, a roadless campground with outhouse, adding 1.4 miles to your trek. The entire lakeshore loop covers 7.5 miles.

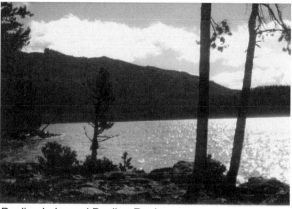

Paulina Lake and Paulina Peak

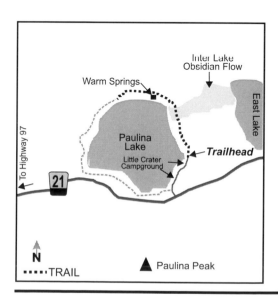

TRAIL CONDITION
mostly smooth, some roots & rocks

TRAILHEAD FACILITIES
outhouse nearby

EXPOSURE
shaded and open

USE

moderate

NOTES
Trekking poles helpful for optional section; mosquitoes likely in mid-summer.

TIDBITS

On his 2nd expedition through Central Oregon in November of 1826, Peter Skeen Ogden discovered East and Paulina Lakes. The latter is named after Walapi Chief Paulina. Both lakes were formed, originally as one, when 10,000' Mt Newberry erupted and collapsed. A later lava flow divided the lake in two.

WALK

The Dry Forest

27 miles
to
Bend

Water
Forest
Meadow
(View)

This is a marvelous short outing for anyone, but *Walkers* and some *Strollers* will especially appreciate the opportunity to venture into the wilderness on a relatively smooth, level trail. The short trip takes you through an airy forest and small lava flow and ends in a grassy meadow edged by Soda Creek. *Strollers* will want a trekking pole or walking companion for assistance on several short stretches that are somewhat steep and rocky. This trail is much less crowded than the Green Lakes Trail just to the west, but you're likely to encounter a few hikers and horses.

Getting there

- *Drive west from Bend on Highway 46/Century Drive, driving 4.5 miles past Mt Bachelor Ski Resort.*
- *Turn right into the Green Lakes Trail parking area.*
- *Find the Soda Creek trailhead on the right (east) side of the parking area. Fill out the free wilderness permit.*

MILES
2.5 - 4.5

ELEV. GAIN
150 - 350'

PERMIT
NW Forest Pass

OPEN
*July to
October/
November*

MAPS
Geo Graphics **Three Sisters Wilderness Map**, Deschutes National Forest Map, USGS **Broken Top**.

The trail sets off through a narrow, uphill trough. The first three–eighths mile is the hardest on this trip, with some roots and rocks to avoid. The path then levels out to a very nice pumice surface with just a few roots and very gradual ups and downs. Through the trees to the left, you'll start to notice views of South Sister with its glaciers. Soon after, the highest points of Broken Top become visible, steep and bare on their south facing sides. As you walk farther through the dry lodgepole forest, mountain hemlocks and a few subalpine firs appear among the pines. Peculiar rock ridges and formations border the trail in places. Stroll through a sunny, open area where lava flowed centuries ago, then step into a forest of older mountain hemlocks just before dropping into the peaceful, stream–edged meadow. There's a nice picnic spot along the creek to the right of your path. Continue forward on the trail to find other lunch and meadow–view sites.

If you want a bit more exercise, you can walk to a rushing cascade upstream on Soda Creek. Follow the trail as it skirts around the meadow, ford a tributary on large rocks, then cross a dry creek bed. After a time you'll cross Crater Creek and enter a noticeably older and cooler forest of stately hemlocks and firs. Listen for the sound of rushing water as you walk through a small sloped meadow then into the forest again. Finally, you'll step into a sunny creek basin with tumbled rocks. The stream cascades down and around a tall basalt bluff which marks the turnaround point for this outing. (*Adventure Hikers* can continue, turning right to go to Todd Lake, 9 miles round trip, or turning left to visit Green Lakes, a 12 mile loop; be sure to use your *Three Sisters Wilderness* map.)

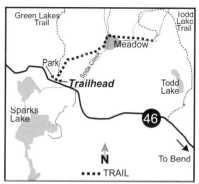

Walk back to Soda Creek, taking time to enjoy the meadow before heading to your car. You'll know you are near the trailhead when you see views ahead of Mt. Bachelor.

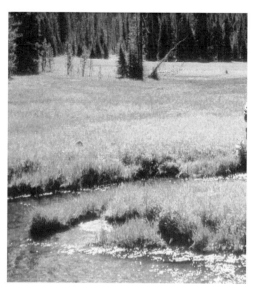

Soda Creek and the meadow

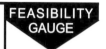

FEASIBILITY GAUGE

TRAIL CONDITION
mostly smooth, some roots & rocks

TRAILHEAD FACILITIES
outhouse

EXPOSURE
airy forest

USE
🚶 🐴
moderate

NOTES
Trekking poles helpful for short steeper section; mosquitoes likely in mid-summer.

TIDBITS

The Deschutes National Forest is home to 182,740 acres of wilderness distributed among five areas — Three Sisters, Mt. Jefferson, Mt. Washington, Thielsen and Diamond Peak. Trail work in the wilderness is done with handsaws and hand drills. Trails are open to hikers and horses but not mountain bikes.

WALK

FACT FINDER

The Waterfall Feast

*Formerly Squaw Creek Falls

37 miles to Bend

Water
Forest
Geology

Waterfall and forest lovers will appreciate this short outing. *Walkers* may want to stop at the first falls, while *Hikers* will enjoy continuing to the third falls. The sound of fast–moving water is a pleasant accompaniment along a good part of the trail. Tree identification provides an interesting challenge; you'll have opportunity to practice distinguishing between spruce and fir trees (see Appendix A for help).

Getting there

- *Drive 8 miles south from Sisters on Road 16 (Elm St.).*
- *Turn west (right) on Rd 1514 and drive 5 miles.*
- *Turn left on Rd 600 and drive about 2 miles. This is a narrow, rocky road, but a car can negotiate it slowly.*
- *Turn left on Rd 680. The road ends in 0.3 mile at the trailhead. Fill out the wilderness permit.*

MILES
1.5 – 3.0

ELEV. GAIN
150 – 300'

PERMIT
NW Forest Pass

OPEN
July to October/ November

MAPS
Geo Graphics *Three Sisters Wilderness Map*,
Deschutes National Forest Map,
USGS *Broken Top*.

Walk a short distance to the Three Sisters Wilderness sign and on to a log bridge over a creeklet. The trail makes small but steady elevation gains as it winds through a forest of lodgepole and ponderosa pines. Look for a huge dead western white pine as well as mountain hemlocks, subalpine firs, grand firs and Englemann spruces. After about three–fourths mile, you'll reach the first falls where a cleared area makes a nice picnic spot. To the north, catch a glimpse of North Sister's peak. The adventurous (with good knees and backs) can scramble down a small trail to a creek–level viewing site. Whychus Creek fans out and spills over a forty–foot, half–dome cliff to make a wide, dramatic waterfall. In early 2006, The U.S. Board on Geographic Names approved the change from Squaw to Whychus Creek. *Whychus* is a Sahaptin word meaning *the place where we cross the water*.

There are two more falls worth seeing, for those who don't mind following a narrow, sometimes steep and rough trail. Just one–fourth mile past the first falls, the creek tumbles over a short drop at the point where Park Creek flows into Whychus. The trail now literally snakes through the woods for about one–half mile to a rocky, water–level viewpoint for the third falls, which drops grandly through a cliff opening to the boulders below. This is a good turnaround point. For those of you who can't resist going farther for a closer view of the falls, be warned that the unmarked route is steep, slippery with small rocks, and dangerous. Unless you are very fit and have a trekking pole, don't risk this.

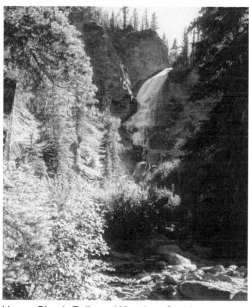

Upper Chush Falls on Whychus Creek

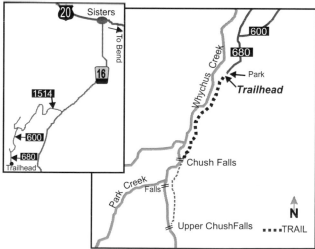

FACT FINDER

IN
Bend

Water Geology Trees

It's hard to believe that such a delightful adventure as this awaits within the city limits of Bend. Like a toddler, the one–minute–peaceful, next–minute–rowdy Deschutes River wins (if not demands) your attention and affection. The awareness of civilization recedes as your senses experience river sounds and forest sights on this short walk along the river's east bank. A new bridge affords the option of combining this trek with *Outing 25* to make a loop instead of an out–and–back.

Getting there

- *From Business Highway 97, turn west on Reed Market Road. (Or take the Reed Market West exit from Highway 97, the Bend Parkway.)*
- *Drive through the circle intersection with Bond Street and Brookswood Boulevard to Farewell Bend Park.*
- *Park near the west end of the park if possible.*

MILES
3

ELEV. GAIN
100'

Find the paved path near the river; walk west past a sandy beach and under the vehicle bridge. Follow the Deschutes River Trail signs. As you walk along near the river bank, take time to read the informational signs posted near the path.

Continuing south, you'll pass some massive ponderosa pines and wind through an assortment of small growth, including bitterbrush, currant and wild roses. Look for vertical basalt walls to the left and a retirement living complex across the river to the right.

PERMIT
none

Shortly, the trail crosses large boulders that might be daunting; some walkers will want trekking poles or a companion to assist them over this section. A long section of boardwalk through dense rushes leads to a view of Central Oregon Irrigation District's hydro site where two buried turbines generate electrical power.

OPEN
all year

Follow the hiker signs at several forks as you begin to gain elevation. Your climb is rewarded when the path levels out with breathtaking views of the churning river and the surprise of a younger, thicker forest.

MAPS
Bend City Map,
USGS *Bend.*

An occasional majestic Douglas fir stands out in contrast. The white-water sounds grow loud again as you approach river level and the new bridge. This is the turn-around point, but if you wish you may cross the river and follow either section of the loop described in *Outing 25*.

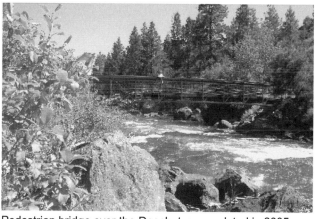

Pedestrian bridge over the Deschutes completed in 2005

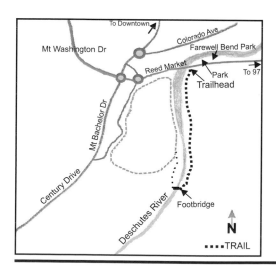

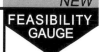
TRAIL CONDITION
smooth, some rocks

TRAILHEAD FACILITIES
restrooms in park

EXPOSURE
mostly shaded

USE
🚶
moderate to heavy

NOTES
Trail can be muddy or snow-packed in winter and spring.

TIDBITS

The Bill Healy Memorial Bridge (you walk under it on this outing) was named for Bend resident Bill Healy who founded the Mt Bachelor Ski Resort in 1958. This award-winning bridge - known as the Southern River Crossing - has a 480' steel plate girder and was designed to complement its canyon setting.

WALK

The Western Movie Set

18 miles
to
Bend

Part of the attraction of Central Oregon is its variety — high desert to the east, mountains and alpine lakes to the west. We recommend taking this walk soon after enjoying one of the mountain outings in order to appreciate the fascinating contrasts that exist within a relatively small area. At times during this unusual trek, you'll feel like you're on a western movie set. Some *Walkers* might find it cumbersome to step over the rocks. You can turn around at almost any point, however, and still feel that you've experienced the flavor of the Dry River Gorge.

Geology
Trees

Getting there

- *Drive east from Bend on Highway 20 (from the traffic light at 27th Street, you'll drive 14.9 miles).*
- *Turn left into a gravel pit area. Drive east around several gravel mounds then down a dirt road winding through rabbit brush toward the juniper trees.*
- *Park about 0.9 miles from the highway in a dirt clearing.*

MILES
4 - 6

ELEV. GAIN
< 50'

PERMIT
none

OPEN
all year

MAPS
Deschutes National Forest Map (trail not marked but follows along the Dry River denoted on map), USGS *Horse Ridge.*

Walk to the east down the dirt road or a small path closer to the highway. You'll soon notice that there seem to be several trails down the gorge; any of them will work. It's impossible to get lost because the high canyon walls keep you funneled in the right direction. The trail is very smooth and dusty in places, but at times you'll have to navigate around or scramble over rocks. The trees here are almost exclusively western juniper, but we counted 4 old growth ponderosa pines. This is one of the few places in the area to see mountain mahogany with its tiny curled leaves and twisted branches; these tree–shrubs range in size from about 15 feet down to small bushes. The high desert brush trio is present here: sage, bitter and rabbit brush; you'll also see some currant.

As you wind through the canyon, watch for shallow cave openings in the high rock wall to your left and later to the right. We spotted an eagle's nest in the columnar basalt cliffs about one mile into the walk. The cliff walls and rimrock, with their various layers and colors, are fascinating to study; you'll enjoy having binoculars. The rocks and boulders strewn on the canyon floor are dotted with lichens in shades ranging from light green to orange and black. Since lichen can live for centuries, it's fun to imagine ancient residents who may have viewed these same fungus–algae organisms. As you walk up to the first huge ponderosa pine, notice the backdrop of a dramatic cliff wall flecked with chartreuse lichen. For a four mile walk, this is the turn-around point.

If you choose to continue, you'll meander through a charming mahogany–boulder "garden" and on to a place where rocks fill the canyon. We turned around here for a hike of nearly six miles. As you walk back, you can see vehicles traveling along Highway 20 on the rim high to the left. For most of this trek, however, you'd never guess there was a highway overhead.

WALK

Canyon wall above the Dry River

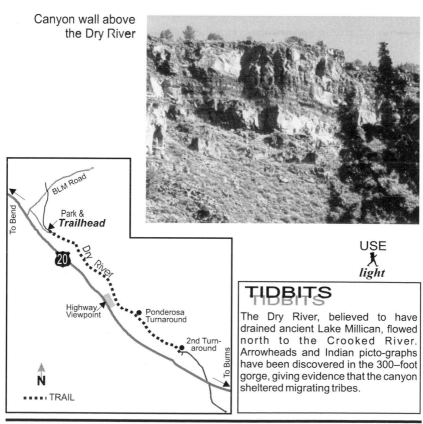

To Bend

BLM Road

Park & **Trailhead**

20

Dry River

Highway Viewpoint

Ponderosa Turnaround

2nd Turn-around

To Burns

N

▪▪▪▪▪ TRAIL

USE
light

TIDBITS

The Dry River, believed to have drained ancient Lake Millican, flowed north to the Crooked River. Arrowheads and Indian picto-graphs have been discovered in the 300–foot gorge, giving evidence that the canyon sheltered migrating tribes.

45 miles to Bend

View
Water
Forest
Geology

Getting there

- Drive west from Sisters on Highway 20 for 12.4 miles to a sign for Mt. Jefferson Wilderness Trailheads.
- Turn right (north) and follow Road 12 for 4 miles.
- Turn left onto paved Road 1230 and drive 1.6 miles.
- Turn left onto gravel Road 1234 and drive 1 mile to a sign for Jack Lake Trailheads.
- Turn left onto a cinder road. Drive 5 miles to a gravel parking area.

MILES
4.4

ELEV. GAIN
200'

PERMIT
NW Forest Pass

OPEN
July to October/ November

MAPS
Geo Graphics **Mt Jefferson Wilderness Map**, Deschutes National Forest Map, USGS **Marion Lake.**

Here's a non–threatening wilderness walk with starting point at pretty little Jack Lake and turn–around point at picturesque Wasco. In between, you can expect a fascinating variety of healthy and burned forest land as well as mountain views and a waterfall treat on sparkling Canyon Creek.

Near the north end of the parking lot, a sign points right to Canyon Glacier Trail #4010. Walk toward Jack Lake and a sign–in board and fill out a wilderness permit. The trail follows around the northeast side of Jack Lake through a forest of subalpine firs plus ponderosa and lodgepole pines. Manzanita and fern compete for space on the forest floor where mountain hemlock and grand fir trees soon outnumber the pines. At the wilderness sign, walk to the right.

This section of trail meanders in and out of forest burned in the B & B Complex fire of 2003. Charred trees contrast starkly with the beargrass, huckleberry and wildflowers beneath them. One benefit of the thinned forest is the mountain views. Watch for Mt. Jefferson to the right and Three Fingered Jack to the left.

When the trail reaches a junction, stay on the low path to your right. A sign points to Wasco Lake. Walk to Canyon Creek and enjoy the lovely two–tiered waterfall. Cross on the halved–log footbridge. The trail now meanders along a ledge with gradual ups and downs. You'll pass through some forested area that's charred and some that's only partially burned. If you walk in late July, you'll enjoy abundant wildflowers, including lupine, fireweed, penstemon and columbine. We even saw bleeding heart in one drainage ditch. Look for several mini–lakes with grassy banks down to the right.

At Wasco choose a spot near the lake for pictures and perhaps lunch. As you leave, notice the boulder–strewn bank west of the lake. Follow the same path back to Jack Lake, watching for Black Butte in the distance as you approach the lake.

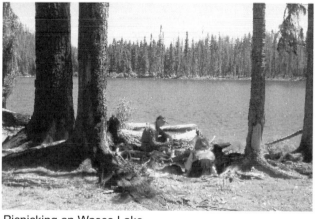

Picnicking on Wasco Lake

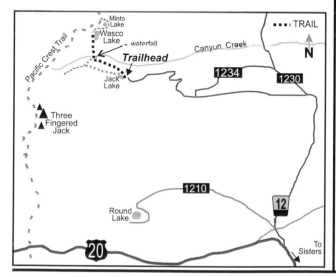

FEASIBILITY GAUGE

TRAIL CONDITION
some roots & rocks

TRAILHEAD FACILITIES
outhouse, tables

EXPOSURE
partly shaded

USE
🚶 🐎
moderate

NOTES
Some folks may not like the log bridge over Can-yon Creek. Mosquitoes likely in late summer.

TIDBITS
The name Wasco most likely comes from the Indian tribe bearing that name. It was a Chinook tribe who lived in north central Oregon. The word was shortened from *wiss-co-pam* or *wasco-pam*, meaning *makers of basins*. The Wasco Indians made elabo-rately carved bowls of horn.

WALK

FACT FINDER

The Enchanted River

41 miles to Bend

Water
Forest
Meadow

Frothy whitewater, quiet green pools and cascading springs beckon you to these charming river trails set in a forest of remarkable variety. Having a state fish hatchery as a staging area is a bonus. You'll want to save time to stroll among the fish tanks and ponds after the trek. *Hikers* might elect to do both trails in one outing. *Walkers* will want to choose one, then come another day and do the other. The trails are relatively smooth, with just a few small rocks and roots and some muddy spots. The Camp Sherman store makes a nice refreshment stop after your outing, and if there's still time left, be sure to visit the Head of the Metolius (*Outing 3*).

Getting there

- *Drive west from Sisters on Highway 20 almost 10 miles to a sign for Camp Sherman and the Metolius River.*
- *Turn right (north) on Road 14 and drive just over 10 miles (Rd 14 curves east then back north and passes several campgrounds), to a sign for Wizard Falls Fish Hatchery.*
- *Turn left and cross the river into the parking area.*

MILES
North – 6
South – 5.4

ELEV. GAIN
North – <75'
South – <100'

PERMIT
none

OPEN
May to December

MAPS
Deschutes National Forest Map, USGS *Candle Creek.*

To walk the **north trail**, head down to the river from any part of the fish hatchery, find the path and turn left. For most of this route, your constant companion is the Metolius River, wending its way toward the Deschutes, becoming en route a swollen finger of Lake Billy Chinook. There's plenty of river life to observe, with various trout (sometimes you can spot them), waterfowl, lush foliage along the banks, and a few anglers. After about a mile, most folks will want to turn left and follow the main path as it skirts around a private meadow. (It's possible to stay next to the river through this section, but the trail, muddy and faint at times, will lead you through some stretches of dense foliage.) We especially enjoyed the forest along the river's banks. In addition to the customary firs and ponderosa pines, watch for Douglas–fir, with three–pronged bracts on its cone, and incense cedar, with its peculiar little duck–bill cone. We also spotted a few western larch trees, easily identified by the way the 2" needles cluster on knobby bases along the twig and also by the yellow color in fall.

The trail rejoins the river and continues downstream to Lower Bridge Campground. At this point, you can return the way you came or cross the bridge and follow the path along the east side, skirting some private land and passing through two campgrounds.

The **south trail** begins where the parking area meets the forest. Head upstream through a dry forest above the river. In just over half a mile look for islands in midstream, then a series of white water rapids that challenge rafters (we enjoyed this thrilling excursion several years ago). You'll cross a segment of trail muddied by springs, then pass through a canyon with stately ponderosa pines. In about 2.5 miles, watch the far riverbank for a pretty postcard scene of mysterious springs cascading down mossy rocks and joining the river. The trail arrives in another quarter mile at a campground where Canyon Creek, bloated from the additions of Roaring and Brush Creeks, joins the Metolius. This is a picturesque spot to enjoy lunch. As you retrace your steps back to the fish hatchery, you're sure to observe some of nature's wonders that you missed the first time.

Metolius River

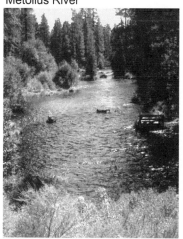

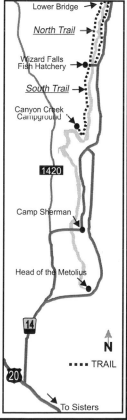

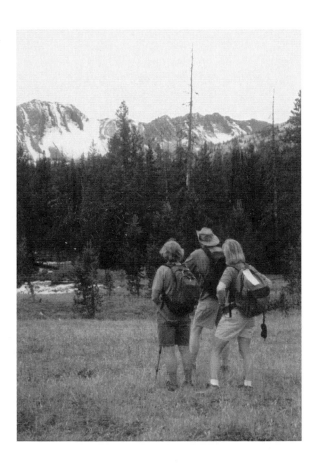

Now it's time for the meat course. You'll find everything here from a delicate poached fish to hearty and messy barbeque ribs. Is the food analogy a bit confusing? What we mean to say is that we've offered several levels of longer outings. Some are flat and others are steep. A few trails are smooth, a few quite rocky. We've classified several hikes as adventure outings; they're for the gutsy and very fit hiker. We only wish the written word could adequately express the delight we felt on each and every trek.

HIKES

Part Four

FACT FINDER

48 miles to Bend

Forest Water Geology

If you're in a tropical mood, this magical outing is for you. Located on the western tip of our 50–mile radius, the trail passes through a greater variety of deciduous foliage than any other hike we describe. There are no views of snow–clad peaks, and the lake, while charming, is no more remarkable than many other alpine beauties. It's the getting there that's the rewarding experience — a sumptuous treat for *Hikers* and fit *Walkers*. *Adventure Hikers* might appreciate scrambling up to a splendid waterfall above the lake.

Getting there

- *Drive west from Sisters on Highway 242 to McKenzie Pass.*
- *Continue down the other side about 11.5 miles to Alder Springs Campground, just past milepost 67.*
- *Park on the right (this area can be crowded); the trailhead is across the road. Fill out a free wilderness permit.*

MILES
3.8 – 4.8

ELEV. GAIN
300 - 450'

PERMIT
NW Forest Pass

OPEN
June/July to October

MAPS
Geo Graphics *Three Sisters Wilderness Map*, Willamette National Forest Map, USGS *Linton Lake*.

The first mile takes you through a forest of mountain hemlock and Douglas–fir trees with giant rhododendron shrubs sprinkled in. The path meanders up a lava flow with draws and gullies of tumbled, mossy lava rock falling away to either side. Vine maple growing in the lava is chartreuse in the summer sun and bright shades of red to yellow in the fall. The magical moment of this hike comes after you crest the lava ridge and turn a sharp corner, switchbacking down into "wonderland." It's not hard to imagine yourself in another time and place here. The old growth Douglas–firs and western redcedars will take your breath away. It seems like quite a descent, especially noting the massive rock bank to the left. However, it's really not bad climbing back out on the return trip. When you see turquoise through the trees, you'll know Linton Lake is near. The path stays high above the lake, then drops down to Obsidian Creek and a small sandy beach. We once carried a rubber boat in to the lake and enjoyed paddling around the perimeter.

The *Adventure Hiker* who has good knees, back and heart might consider going to the waterfall on Linton

Creek. Cross Obsidian Creek (trekking poles really help), then follow a faint path for about one–half mile along the left side of Linton Creek. Each time we go to the falls it seems a bit harder because of more downed trees (the falls trail isn't maintained). The creek makes an eighty–foot plunge that's impressive even late in the season. Follow the same path back down. Don't be tempted to go cross–country to Obsidian Creek and follow it down. We made that mistake only once.

When you hike back out, stop at the last switchback on the high lava ridge and step out to a point on your left. Look back for Linton Falls on the forested slope above the lake.

Falls on Linton Creek

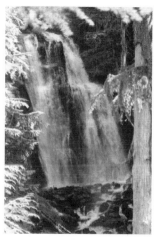

TRAIL CONDITION
some roots & rocks

TRAILHEAD FACILITIES
outhouse

EXPOSURE
mostly shaded

USE
moderate

NOTES
Trekking poles helpful; mosquitoes likely in mid-summer; falls option very steep.

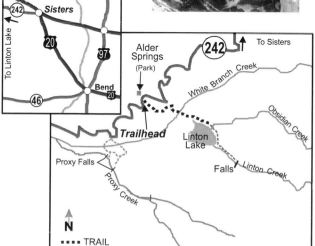

TIDBITS

Linton Lake was formed when a lava flow from Collier Cone dammed Linton Creek. The lake's outlet is an underground flow beneath the lava in Lost Creek Canyon. Linton Falls, high above the lake, spills over a different lava flow.

HIKE

FACT FINDER

35 miles
to
Bend

Forest
Water
Geology

Two glorious alpine lakes, reached via a lovely forest path, are the starring attraction on this short hike or long walk. Plan to spend some time at one or both lakes; hardy souls can take a refreshing dip while others explore along the shorelines. Some *Walkers* may wish to turn around at Blow Lake for an outing of just over 2 miles. Trekking poles will provide extra stability on uphill sections of the trail.

Getting there

- *Drive west from Bend on the Century Drive/Highway 46 about 2 miles past the Elk Lake Resort road on the left to a hiker sign.*
- *Turn right into a parking area. The trailhead is located at the northwest edge of the parking lot. Fill out the free wilderness permit.*

MILES
4.8

ELEV. GAIN
400'

PERMIT
NW Forest Pass

OPEN
*July to
October/
November*

MAPS
Geo Graphics *Three Sisters Wilderness Map*, Deschutes National Forest Map, USGS *Elk Lake.*

Walk through an open lodgepole pine forest sprinkled with subalpine firs and mountain hemlocks. Follow along the left side of a creek bed to a bridge. Cross over and note the steep, rocky banks on the left that give way shortly to green meadow. Soon after crossing a second bridge, look for trails on the right leading to Blow Lake, an alpine beauty with just enough beach for swimming and wading.

Continue on the first trail through a sun–dappled forest with grassy glades along the creek to the left. Bright rays illuminate the yellow–green ground cover and the gray boulders forming low ridges on the right. Just after crossing a stone bridge, look left to see a dramatic gray cliff. One hundred yards after the bridge, walk down to the right to glimpse an unnamed lake. Follow several switchbacks in the trail and look again to the left to see boulders strewn over a high, steep slope. When the trail crests a hill, step to the right and look behind you for a view of Mt. Bachelor. Cross a last needle–covered bridge and begin the final, gradual descent to Doris Lake; side paths lead to this incredible mountain jewel. There are scenic rock peninsulas for lunching and narrow, pebbly beaches suitable for swimming. Take time to enjoy the serenity and charm of the area before retracing your steps to your car. The Elk Lake Resort makes a good refreshment stop on the drive back to Bend.

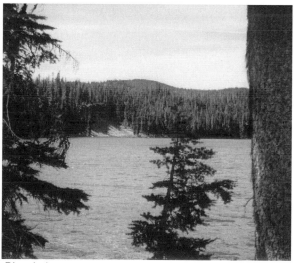

Blow Lake

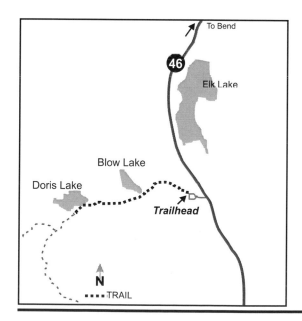

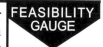
TRAIL
CONDITION
*mostly smooth,
some roots
& rocks*

TRAILHEAD
FACILITIES
outhouse

EXPOSURE
airy forest

USE

*moderate
to heavy*

NOTES
Watch for horses sharing the trail in late summer; mosquitoes likely in mid-summer; swimming optional.

TIDBITS

The Six Lakes Trail continues past Doris Lake to connect with the Pacific Crest Trail, which accesses dozens of wilderness lakes to the west. A left turn at a junction beyond Doris Lake leads to Senoj Lake, 6304' Williamson Mountain, and Lucky Lake, which can also be accessed from a trailhead on Highway 46.

HIKE

40 miles
to
Bend

Spend just half a day and receive immense satisfaction from this short hike along the southern edge of the magnificent Mt. Jefferson Wilderness. The evidence of the B&B Complex fire is more fascinating than distracting. This hike combines nicely with other short outings in the book (such as *outings 3* and *13*) or with shopping in Sisters!

**Water
Forest
Geology**

Getting there

- *Drive west from Sisters on Highway 20 12.4 miles to a sign for Mt. Jefferson Wilderness Trailheads.*
- *Turn right (north) and follow Road 12 for about 1 mile.*
- *Turn left on gravel Road 1210 and drive 5.6 miles.*
- *Turn right on Road 600 (at a sign for a trailhead) and drive 0.6 mile to park. The total distance from Road 12 to parking area is 6.2 miles.*

**MILES
*4.5 +***

**ELEV. GAIN
*450'***

**PERMIT
*NW Forest Pass***

**OPEN
*July to
October/
November***

MAPS
Geo Graphics *Mt
Jefferson Wilderness Map*,*Deschutes
National Forest
Map*, USGS *Three
Fingered Jack.*

The trail starts just above Round Lake and shortly enters the Mt. Jefferson Wilderness. As you traverse along this southern boundary of the wilderness, you may hear an occasional jake brake of an eighteen wheeler descending the Highway 20 grade above Suttle Lake. Much of the lush green forest of pre–fire days has been replaced by charred remains of firs as well as white, ponderosa and lodgepole pines. You'll notice not a few trees shaped like giant peeled bananas, with bark separated from the trunk and curling back to the ground. It's an eerily beautiful scene where a groundcover of beargrass and, appropriately, fireweed is flourishing. Bright green ferns and silvery lupines with blue summer blooms also provide a stunning contrast in the blackened landscape.

The old trail went through a creek bottom close to Long Lake. The new trail stays higher, re–routed due to burned bridges and boardwalks. A few tall green sentinels dot the burned forest, leaving you to wonder why these survivors were so blessed.

The eastern lake shore is composed of gray basalt rocks covered with kinikinick. A few fir and mountain hemlock trees, along with various shrubby plants, have survived near the lake. A rock bluff stands out across the water, and the trail continues on around for those who want to explore the shoreline. It even connects eventually to the Pacific Crest Trail to the west (about a 2.2 mile distance heading southwest from the Booth Lake Trail junction on the north side of Square Lake).

When you're satisfied with your lake explorations, retrace your steps back to the parking area above Round Lake. For a bit more exercise, take time to walk around Round Lake with its gorgeous view of Three Fingered Jack.

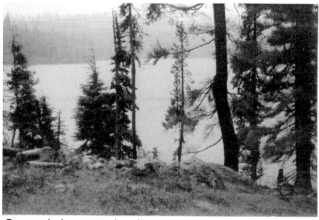

Square Lake on a rainy day

NEW

FEASIBILITY GAUGE

TRAIL CONDITION
some roots & rocks

TRAILHEAD FACILITIES
outhouse, tables nearby at campground

EXPOSURE
mostly open

USE

moderate

NOTES
Mosquitoes likely in late summer. Trekking poles nice for steeper section of trail.

TIDBITS

On August 19, 2003, 2 fires began burning in the Central Oregon Cascades - the Bear Butte fire and the Booth fire. The two burned together on Sept. 4 and became known as the B & B Complex. The fire was contained on Sept. 26 after burning 90,769 acres. Of those acres, 40,419 were burned in the Mt Jefferson Wilderness.

HIKE

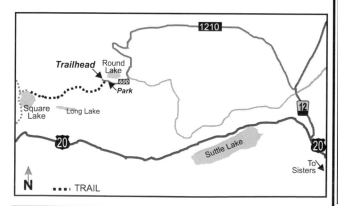

N ····· TRAIL

Meadow View

FACT FINDER

22 miles to Bend

Todd Lake was made for postcards and photo journals! Set in a gorgeous wildflower meadow with views of Mt. Bachelor and Broken Top beyond, you may have a hard time leaving this 45–acre jewel behind. We promise that the views from above plus the additional mountain and meadow vistas will amply reward your efforts. Any in the group who don't wish to climb will be perfectly happy with a short jaunt around the lake.

Forest
View
Water

Getting there

■ *Drive west from Bend on the Century Drive/Highway 46 to the Todd Lake sign (20 miles from the Century/Mt Washington/Reed Market circle).*
■ *Turn right on Road 370 and drive about two-tenths mile to a parking area. Take the path toward the lake and watch for your trailhead to the right.*

MILES
4 +

ELEV. GAIN
550'

The trail gains elevation gradually as you walk through a subalpine fir and hemlock forest that's mostly thick and shady. Keep an eye to the left for views of Mt. Bachelor and Todd Lake and its meadow. A little ways before the 1 mile point you'll cross a creek on a footbridge. Look for a lovely meadow sloping up to your right.

PERMIT
NW Forest Pass

After entering the Three Sisters Wilderness – a sign marks the boundary – the trail traverses an open pumice flat with a stunning view of Broken Top. Look back to see Mt. Bachelor, and when the trail enters the forest again, watch for South Sister ahead.

OPEN
July to October/ November

The pumice flats and the dry grassy meadows that sweep down to the south lend a unique flavor to this hike. Several drainage ditches may overflow early in the season; you'll appreciate waterproof boots if you hike in late June or early July. To take advantage of the wildflower show in the meadows, we would suggest going in mid to late summer.

MAPS
Geo Graphics *Three Sisters Wilderness Map*, Deschutes National Forest Map, USGS *Broken Top.*

Near the two–mile point, the path intersects a trail that winds about 3.7 miles past Soda Creek Meadow to the Green Lakes trailhead. We turned around at this point for a four–mile outing. If you want some more exercise, you can continue straight for just under a mile to reach Cayuse Crater.

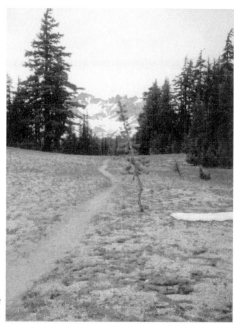

View of
Broken Top

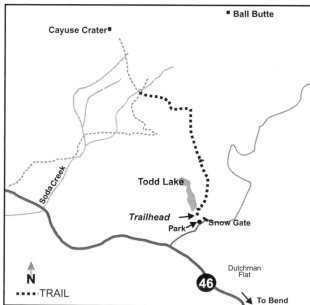

FEASIBILITY
GAUGE

TRAIL
CONDITION
*some rocks
and roots*

TRAILHEAD
FACILITIES
*outhouse,
campground*

EXPOSURE
*part shade,
part open*

USE
🏃 🐎
moderate

NOTES
*Watch for horses
sharing the trail;
trekking poles
nice; mosquitoes
likely in mid-
summer.*

TIDBITS

Originally called Lost Lake, Todd Lake was later renamed so as not to confuse it with other *Lost Lakes* in Oregon. The new name honored John Young Todd who was born in Missouri in 1830 and arrived in Oregon in 1852. He built Sherars Bridge in 1860 and later settled on the Farewell Bend Ranch.

HIKE

In the Shadow of Grandeur

45 miles
to
Bend

View
Water
Forest
Meadow
Geology

You're rewarded before you even start here with a stroll around picturesque little Jack Lake. The walk through a mysterious, varied forest past a couple of surprise ponds adds to your pleasure. The climactic moment comes, however, when you arrive at the meadow and gaze up at rugged Three Fingered Jack. Fit *Walkers* will enjoy this outing along with *Hikers*.

Getting there

- *Drive west from Sisters on Highway 20 for 12.3 miles to a sign, Mt. Jefferson Wilderness Trailheads.*
- *Turn right (north) and follow Road 12 for 4 miles.*
- *Turn left onto paved Road 1230 and drive 1.6 miles.*
- *Turn left onto gravel Road 1234 and drive 1 mile to a sign for Jack Lake Trailheads.*
- *Turn left onto a cinder road. Drive 5 miles to a gravel parking area.*

MILES
4.5

ELEV. GAIN
400'

PERMIT
NW Forest Pass

OPEN
*July to
October/
November*

MAPS
Geo Graphics *Mt
Jefferson Wilder-
ness Map,Deschutes
National Forest
Map,* USGS *Three
Fingered Jack.*

Look for a sign pointing right to Canyon Glacier Trail # 4010. Walk to the sign–in board and fill out a wilderness permit. The trail starts to the right and skirts around the northeast side of Jack Lake through a forest of subalpine firs, ponderosa pines and lodgepole pines. Walk up a small rise into a manzanita and fern "garden." Soon after, you'll enter a park–like setting of mountain hemlock and grand fir trees with dense bear grass carpeting the forest floor. At the Wilderness sign, stay left to walk the loop clockwise. In about one mile, a ridge of massive gray basalt boulders emerges on the right. The trail winds up onto the ridge and soon passes a pond on the left, followed quickly by another, smaller pond. When you walk into an older hemlock and fir forest with very little leafy vegetation, take note of the old man's beard lichen hanging from the trees. After crossing a creek and passing a couple of small meadows, you'll come to the medium–sized Lower Canyon Creek Meadow and a breathtaking view of Three Fingered Jack. It's definitely worth it to continue 0.7 miles to the upper meadow. From that point, the sure-footed may want to traverse 0.8 miles up a steep rocky path to the saddle viewpoint with views beyond Jack to the south.

To continue your loop journey from the lower meadow, find Canyon Creek and a small sign pointing north. The trail leaves the creek about 1/2 mile later and joins the trail from Wasco Lake. At this junction, detour to a footbridge to view a picturesque falls in the creek. Return and head to the left (southeast), walking about 1.5 miles back to your car. When you see Black Butte in the distance and Jack Lake below to the right, you'll know you're nearly there.

FEASIBILITY
GAUGE

Trail to
upper meadow

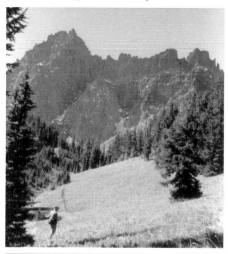

TRAIL CONDITION
many roots & rocks

TRAILHEAD FACILITIES
outhouse, tables

EXPOSURE
mostly shaded

USE
🚶 🐎
moderate

NOTES
Trekking poles helpful in steep, rocky sections; bring binoculars.

TIDBITS

One of the most distinctive volcanos in the area, Three Fingered Jack is a deeply glaciated basaltic andesite shield centered on a pyroclastic cone. Like North Sister and Mt Washington, the 7841' volcano rests on a 10-mile shield base. For a better view, hikers can continue 0.7 mile to the upper meadow.

HIKE

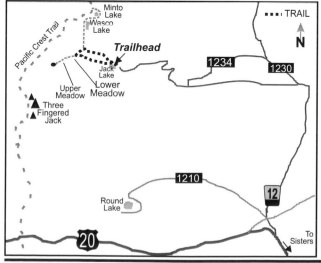

FACT FINDER

21 miles to Bend

View Forest

If you're fairly fit and you love 360–degree views, then this outing is for you. There's no avoiding the steady climb, but the feeling of accomplishment coupled with the postcard panorama will reward you well. We strongly suggest taking trekking poles on this challenging hike. They'll increase your confidence on the steep terrain and provide some help for your knees on the trip down.

Getting there

- *Drive west from Bend 21 miles on Highway 46/Century Drive.*
- *Turn right into the Dutchman Flat Sno-Park.*
- *Don't forget to display your NW Forest Pass.*

MILES 3.5

ELEV. GAIN 1400'

PERMIT NW Forest Pass

OPEN July to November

MAPS
Deschutes National Forest Map, USGS *Broken Top.*

You'll find the trail at the west end of the parking area. This uphill trek allows few breath–catching breaks until you reach the summit. It helps to keep in mind the exhilaration of a panoramic vista awaiting you, and you can use the view behind you as an excuse for short rest stops. Although it's steep, the fairly smooth trail meanders through a pleasant forest of subalpine firs and mountain hemlocks. Several grassy mini–meadows provide a sunny contrast to the woods. Your final assault on the peak is steeper yet, with some loose scree. Trekking poles are definitely helpful here.

The broad, fairly flat top of the mountain affords a fun diversion for map lovers. Look back to the south to pick out Edison Butte and Kwolh Butte, both east of Mt. Bachelor. Walk north past the foundation of a long–gone lookout tower and find the Swampy Lakes meadow and the city of Bend to the east. Follow the cinder path to the highest point on the west side of the crest. From here you'll see Sparks Lake, South and Middle Sisters and Broken Top.

Walk carefully back down the steep, loose section of trail, then enjoy the expansive southern views as you continue to the base. If you have your binoculars, you can search for hikers or lift–riders on Mt. Bachelor.

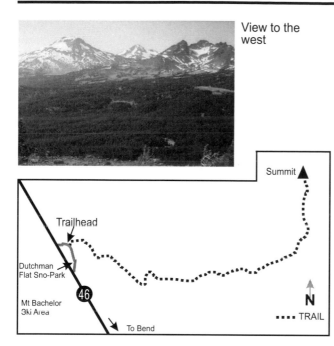

View to the west

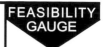
Summit

Trailhead

Dutchman
Flat Sno-Park

Mt Bachelor
Ski Area

46

To Bend

N

•••• TRAIL

TRAIL CONDITION
mostly smooth, some roots & rocks

TRAILHEAD FACILITIES
outhouse

EXPOSURE
part shaded, part open

USE
light

NOTES
Trekking poles helpful; steep hike; bring binoculars.

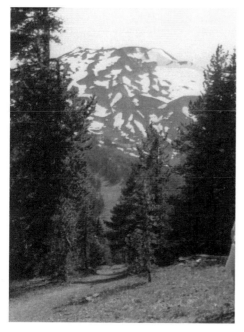

View of Mt Bachelor to the south

TIDBITS

Air cools at about four degrees Farenheit per 1000–foot elevation gain. At 7,775', Tumalo Mountain's summit temperature should be about 16 degrees cooler than Bend's temperature.

HIKE

Oasis Under the Rimrock

FACT FINDER

29 miles
to
Bend

Water
Geology
View

This excursion provides a desert serendipity — the surprise of a deep creek canyon seemingly falling out the bottom of the desert plateau. You'll enjoy the micro climates of the dramatic canyon and of an adjacent gulch with bubbling springs. Rattlesnakes have been known to frequent the creek banks in summer. We suggest taking this hike in fall when the temperature has dropped and the snakes have gone to bed. Fit *Walkers* might enjoy all or parts of this outing along with the *Hikers*. We recommend trekking poles for several steep sections of trail.

Getting there

- *Drive west from Bend on Highway 20 (drive 10.5 miles from the intersection in north Bend of Highways 97 and 20).*
- *Turn right (north) on Fryrear Road and drive just over 6 miles to an intersection with Highway 126. Cross 126 and continue on Holmes Road almost 7 miles to Road 6360 on the left. This is easy to miss, but it's just opposite milepost 7.*
- *Drive north on this gravel road 4 miles to a sign for Alder Springs Trailhead.*
- *Turn right (east) onto a dirt road and drive about 0.8 miles to a parking area.*

MILES
4.6

ELEV. GAIN
350'

PERMIT
none

OPEN
April –
December

MAPS
Deschutes National Forest Map,
USGS *Steelhead Falls.*

Walk to the trailhead at the east side of the parking lot. The dirt path runs north and east for 0.3 miles to a trail junction just past a power–line pole. Stay to the right and follow along the east side of Whychus Creek Canyon, noting occasional views of the creek with tall ponderosa pines on the banks. The path takes a big step up onto table rock then passes through a barren area with several rock cairns marking the way. After crossing an old dirt road, turn right at a juniper tree and wind down into a smaller creek canyon. You'll cross the usually dry creek, and continue down the gulch through juniper trees, bunch grass, sagebrush, bitterbrush and rabbit brush. A few ponderosas grace the landscape as you descend, and the cliff walls, with their colorful striations, demand your attention. Soon after you hear gurgling water, turn down a faint side trail to the left and explore along the unnamed creek. Follow the stream south to see Alder Springs bubbling out of the rocks. When you rejoin the main trail, look for a short, rocky path on the right that leads you into a unique half–barrel–like rock formation with water–washed bowls on its walls. The secrets of the high desert never cease to amaze us! The main trail leads shortly to a meadow oasis edged by Whychus Creek (formerly Squaw) to the north and the unnamed creek to the west. On your right, another creek flows into Whychus just before it intersects the cliff wall and turns abruptly north.

After enjoying this creek–side steppe, start back up the main trail. As you climb out of the smaller gulch onto the rim of Whychus Creek Canyon, look to the west and south for panoramic Cascade views. When you reach the trail junction near the power pole, follow a faint trail to the right that takes you in about one–half mile to the canyon edge above Whychus Creek. You can walk to the south a short distance, then walk north down to creek level. There's a pretty, grassy picnic spot here. Continue north between the creek and the cliff about one–fourth mile to a ponderosa "gate." You might go a bit farther on flat, layered rocks jutting into the water. As you walk back, enjoy the color variety of the cliff walls.

Walkers who prefer a shorter outing can omit Alder Springs and hike only to Whychus Creek. This portion totals about 1.6 miles (plus 0.6 to explore along the creek) and about 200' elevation gain.

TRAIL CONDITION
some rocky places

TRAILHEAD FACILITIES
none

EXPOSURE
open

USE
light

NOTES
Trekking poles helpful; you might see a rattlesnake in summer.

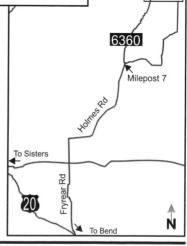

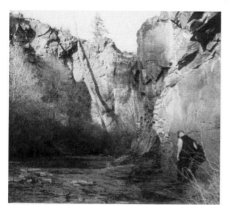

Whychus Creek Canyon

HIKE

4 miles
to
Bend

Water
Forest
Geology

"So close and yet so far away!" That's how you'll feel in Shevlin Park, a year–round oasis just west of Bend. In a couple of hours you'll experience the charred landscape left by the 1990 Awbrey Hall fire, a lush creek canyon, and a typical Central Oregon hillside. Locals and tourists love the park, but most stay in the picnic areas near the creek. Expect to encounter a few hikers and some mountain bikers on the rim trail. This makes a fine outing for wintertime when many trails are covered with snow.

Getting there

- *Drive west on Greenwood Avenue from its intersection with Third St. (Business 97) in Bend.*
- *Continue west as Greenwood becomes Newport and finally Shevlin Park Road (about 4 miles total).*
- *Cross Tumalo Creek and turn left into a parking area at the Shevlin Park gate.*

MILES
4.7

ELEV. GAIN
300 '

PERMIT
none

OPEN
all year
can be muddy
or snow-packed
in winter/spring

MAPS
*USGS **Shevlin Park**,*
Deschutes National
Forest Map.

Just past the entrance gate, walk left through an aspen grove and a meadow to the footbridge over Tumalo Creek. Follow the trail up a burned slope, then turn south and continue along the ridge. Recent undergrowth of bunch grass plus bitterbrush, currant and manzanita join ponderosa pines that survived the fire. The trail coincides with a dirt road for a quarter mile before dropping down into the green creek canyon. If you hike in fall, you can easily identify the western larches that grow here by the gold color of their needles. A right–hand fork takes you down to an enchanting "garden" of massive boulders and ancient ponderosas. Cross a footbridge over a side stream and climb back up to the canyon rim.

The trail meanders past basalt outcroppings and drops into a darker forest of subalpine firs, some Douglas–firs and even a few Englemann spruces. You will cross Tumalo Creek on a renovated log bridge (don't fret — it has handrails), then cross a dirt road and veer right up a sloped path edged with snowbrush. As you walk back northeast toward the entrance gate, notice Fremont meadow across the road to the right. This side of the canyon is much drier, and juniper trees soon appear among the ponderosas and manzanita. You will pass a trail leading to the covered bridge at

Hixon Crossing, a supply road (the trail jogs right here), and a road winding up Red Tuff Gulch, before meeting the park road near the ranger cottage. Turn left on the park road and walk the short distance to the parking area.

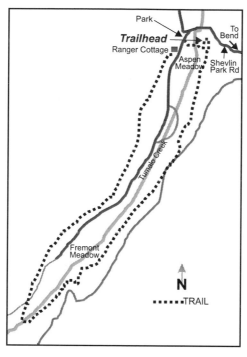

FEASIBILITY GAUGE

TRAIL CONDITION
some rocks & roots

TRAILHEAD FACILITIES
outhouse, tables (in park)

EXPOSURE
part open, part shaded

USE
heavy

NOTES

Trekking poles helpful for steeper sections; mosquitoes likely in midsummer.

TIDBITS

The land for Shevlin Park was donated by the Shevlin-Hixon Company in memory of Thomas L. Shevlin, the company's first president. The area was "discovered" by the Fremont party in December of 1843. In 1929 the city acquired the Tumalo Fish Hatchery, previously abandoned by the state because the creek often froze in winter.

HIKE

Balancing rock in Red Tuff Gulch

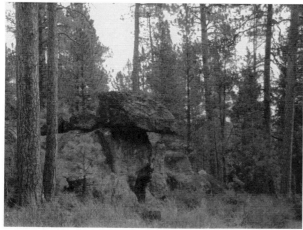

16 miles
to
Bend

Geology
View
Forest

While this is not the first outing we would re-commend to visitors, it is noteworthy for its unusual rock formations. The reward for a rather mundane trek through sandy desert is the adventure of exploring the natural rock fortresses. Marsha's husband described these after flying over the area, and we knew we had to see them up close. We weren't disappointed. This is an easy outing for *Hikers*; many *Walkers* will also enjoy it.

Getting there

- *Drive east from Bend on Highway 20 to milepost 16.*
- *Turn left (north) into a parking area.*
- *Pick up a map at the information board.*

MILES
6 - 8

ELEV. GAIN
< 100'

PERMIT
none

OPEN
all year

MAPS
Badlands Interim Travel Map avail-able at trailhead. USGS Horse Ridge and Alfalfa.

Walk to the right, or east, down a dirt road which curves and heads north. Stay on this main trail, avoid-ing five paths to the east and two that head back to the west and south. The vegetation here is almost exclu-sively sagebrush, bunch grass and juniper. The trail, dusty in summer, passes through some sections of rocky ground. The sparse juniper forest provides a transition between the sagebrush desert to the east and the forested mountains to the west. Studying the juniper trees, each with its own quirky character, makes an interesting diversion. Some look like domestic shrubs, others like gnarled oldsters who've witnessed more than their share of wind, weather and life. Western juniper can live for hundreds of years, and you'll see some fine grandpapas here.

After walking nearly three miles, you'll come to a right–turn trail junction with a large rock formation to the left. Allow half an hour or so to explore this fas-cinating fortress. We walked a short distance north around it and scrambled over some rocks to get "inside." As you investigate, you'll find two layers of narrow, sandy–floored canyons forming a horseshoe around a high juniper–and–sage plateau. Watch for shallow cave openings, wind–eroded pockets in the rock walls, and evidence of bird nests and bat hideouts. Can't you just visualize ancient peoples fending off enemies from this rocky stronghold? Make your way to the plateau for sweeping mountain views: Horse Ridge to the south, the Maury Mountains and the Ochocos to the east, Mt. Hood to the north, following around to Jefferson, Three Fingered Jack, Washington, the Three Sisters and Broken Top.

Go back to the trail and walk east one–half mile to reach the second fortress, similar to the first but more circular in shape. We entered on the north, climbing up a mossy gully. On the east side there are multiple layers of canyons or cracks, some with narrow openings to the outside. Watch your footing here; there are steep drop–offs and sections that could break down under your weight. If you look to the east from here, you'll see Badlands Rock, shaped like a rough pyramid that collapsed in on itself. It can be reached by hiking another half mile east on the trail. When you've finished exploring, walk back to the trail junction and head south along the same route to the parking area.

FEASIBILITY GAUGE

TRAIL CONDITION
mostly smooth, some rocks

TRAILHEAD FACILITIES
none

EXPOSURE
open

USE
🚶 🚴 🐎
light

NOTES
This is a good cool-season outing.

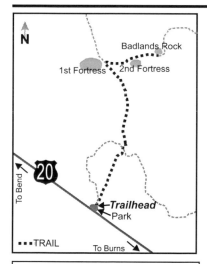

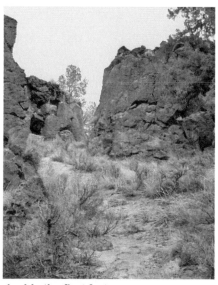

Inside the first fortress

TIDBITS The basalt pressure ridges of Badlands are considered recent volcanic activity in the Brothers fault zone. The juniper forest is one of the world's largest stands of western juniper.

HIKE

FACT FINDER

Nature's Swimming Resort

43 miles to Bend

Water
Forest
View
Geology

You'll not want to miss this delightful hike which takes you past gorgeous Benson Lake to our favorite Cascade Lakes. Tenas Lakes are green jewels set into gray cliffs and rocky shores. You'll enjoy the adventure of treasure–hunting for each jewel, and, if hiking on a hot day, you'll want to wear your swimsuit under your hiking clothes. This is a fairly easy outing for *Hikers*; fit *Walkers* will be amply rewarded, even though the length and elevation gain here are greater than most WALKS. You'll find trekking poles an asset on steeper trail segments.

Getting there

- *Drive west from Sisters on McKenzie Highway 242.*
- *Drive 5.6 miles west of McKenzie Pass to a hiker sign near Scott Lake.*
- *Turn right (north) and drive 1.5 miles to the trailhead.*
- *Fill out a free wilderness permit.*

MILES 5

ELEV. GAIN 700'

PERMIT NW Forest Pass

OPEN June/July to October

MAPS
Geo Graphics *Mt Washington Wilderness Map*, *Deschutes National Forest Map*, USGS *Linton Lake*.

Begin hiking to the west on trail #3502. The forest here consists of mountain hemlocks and lodgepole pines, plus subalpine and grand firs with a bear grass carpet. Also watch for western white pines with their longer cones. At just under a mile, you'll cross the outlet creek, dry in late summer, that runs from Benson to Scott Lake. At 1.4 miles, look for a trail leading to Benson Lake on the left. Postpone your exploration of Benson and continue on past a still pond to the left and a "puddle" on the right. Keep watching for views of Benson through the trees. The Tenas trail passes several small meadows, then switchbacks across boulder–strewn slopes. This, to us, is the ultimate in natural landscaping — it's what we would do on our properties if we could. After passing a tiny lake, you'll walk through two open areas with meager vegetation and come to a small wooden sign pointing left to Tenas Lakes.

The first peanut–shaped lake is the largest. This is a wonderful swimming lake with a small gravelly beach on the trail side and many large, smooth boulders for sun drying when you come out; towels are optional. If there are already folks here, you're sure to find solitude at one of the other lakes. There are three medium–sized lakes good for swimming, one to the south and two to the west, plus several small or tiny lakes. Part of the joy of this outing is to "discover" all the lakes. Our favorite is the medium lake to the northwest with its cliff backdrop. If you choose to scramble up the bluff north of this lake, you'll be rewarded with far–reaching views of foothills and valleys to the west, Scott Mountain to the north, and the Three Sisters and The Husband to the southeast. One challenge of this outing is selecting a site to picnic or contemplate the beauty. There are just too many lovely spots.

On the return trip take time to explore Benson Lake, a stunner in its own right, whose only misfortune was to be placed so close to the Tenas beauty queens. Go around the lake to the left on a faint trail up a high ridge. You'll find views of the lake below and then a panoramic vista point taking in Mt. Washington, the crater peaks of Belknap, Little Belknap and Black, plus the snow caps of the Three Sisters and The Husband. Walk back down the way you came up, then turn right on the main trail and head to your car.

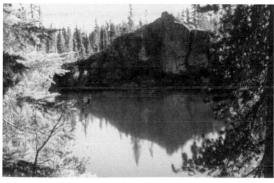

One of the Tenas Lakes

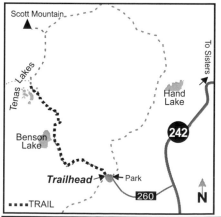

FEASIBILITY GAUGE

TRAIL CONDITION
some roots & rocks

TRAILHEAD FACILITIES
outhouse

EXPOSURE
shaded

USE
🚶 🐎
moderate to heavy

NOTES
Mosquitoes likely in mid-summer; swimming optional.

TIDBITS

The Mt Washington Wilderness covers 52,516 acres along the Cascade crest. 28 lakes can be found here, including Benson, Tenas, and Hand, which was formed when lava from Twin Craters dammed an outlet. 6616-foot Scott Mountain, a shield volcano, makes for a good extension of the Tenas hike. The trek to the summit and back will add 2.2 miles to the outing.

HIKE

**43 miles
to
Bend**

**Water
Forest
View**

Hikers and fit *Walkers* will enjoy the magic of the varied forests on this outing. After passing through a park–like grassy woodland, you'll descend into an older, cooler forest — home to the Patjens Lakes. You'll then view large blue Big Lake through the filter of mature hemlocks and firs. You'll also be treated to some lovely mountain views and a pleasant, sandy beach. The challenge for *Walkers* will come in the one–half mile uphill stretch near the beginning of the trek and in the overall length of the loop.

Getting there

- *Drive west from Sisters on Highway 20 and turn south at the sign for Hoodoo Ski Area.*
- *Drive 4 miles on Big Lake Road to a hiker sign and trail-head on the right (just past West Big Lake Campground).*
- *Fill out the permit for the Mt. Washington Wilderness.*

**MILES
6**

**ELEV. GAIN
400'**

**PERMIT
NW Forest Pass**

**OPEN
July/Aug
to October/
November**

MAPS
Geo Graphics *Mt Washington Wilderness Map*,
Willamette National
Forest Map,
USGS *Clear Lake.*

Walk 0.1 mile to a fork and go to the right to start the loop trail. The great numbers of bear grass clumps lend this forest of lodgepole pines and subalpine firs a landscaped feel. As you progress, you'll note more and more mountain hemlock trees. The trail parallels a sunny creek glade on the left, then starts a gradual climb. After a short dip, you'll start climbing in earnest. Be prepared to gain most of this trip's elevation in the next one–half mile. Look to the right for views through the trees of Sand Mountain, a basaltic cinder cone with a lookout tower on one of its two humps. As you top the crest, watch for North Sister straight ahead with Middle and South Sisters just beyond. The trail enters the Mt. Washington Wilderness just as Mt. Washington becomes visible.

As you make a long gradual descent, you'll pass through several sloped bracken meadows and an enchanting mixed forest. Look now for western white pines and Douglas–firs. The trail seems to wind down into a deep valley (yes, you will have to gain back some of this elevation, but not all). Watch for the first small and shallow Patjens Lake on the right. Continue about three–eighths mile to the second lake on the left. In low–water years, these lakes are surrounded by grass meadows. The third lake is the largest; the fourth is often just a puddle in late summer.

From the fourth lake, you'll hike just under 1.5 miles back to Big Lake (take the fork to the left). The secluded beach on south Big Lake is a nice place to rest, wade or swim. Walk another one mile, passing through stately hemlocks and an almost pure stand of subalpine firs, back to the parking area. Look for imposing Mt. Washington southeast of the lake.

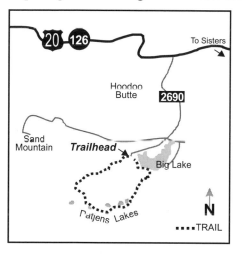

Largest Patjens Lake

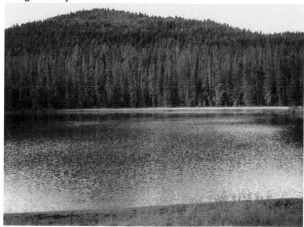

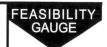

FEASIBILITY GAUGE

TRAIL CONDITION
mostly smooth, some roots & rocks

TRAILHEAD FACILITIES
outhouse

EXPOSURE
shaded

USE
🚶 🐎
moderate to heavy

NOTES
Trekking poles helpful for short steeper section; mosquitoes in mid-summer; swimming optional.

TIDBITS

The Sand Mountain Volcanic field is made up of twenty cinder cones, including Twin Craters, Nash and Little Nash Craters. Patjens Lakes received their name from Henry Patjens, a Grass Valley sheep rancher who brought flocks to summer pasture near the lakes.

HIKE

36 miles to Bend

Water
View
Forest
Geology

This delightful hike has it all — majestic views, awe–inspiring forests, jewel–like lakes and interesting volcanic formations. In short, it's the perfect Central Oregon representative experience. It's a fairly easy outing for *Hikers* and a challenging outing (because of length and elevation gain) for *Walkers*. There's a small section where the slope drops steeply away from the trail; however, the path is comfortably wide. Trekking poles will provide extra security.

Getting there

- *Drive west from Sisters on McKenzie Highway 242.*
- *Just before McKenzie Pass and about 14.5 miles from Sisters, turn left to Lava Camp Lake.*
- *Follow this cinder road for about 0.5 mile and turn right to the Pacific Crest Trail parking area.*
- *Fill out a free wilderness permit.*

**MILES
6**

**ELEV. GAIN
800'**

**PERMIT
*NW Forest Pass***

**OPEN
*July/Aug
to October/
November***

MAPS
Geo Graphics *Three Sisters Wilderness Map*, Deschutes National Forest Map, USGS *North Sister*.

Take the path on the right (west) which directs you to the PCNST (Pacific Crest National Scenic Trail). When you reach the PCT in about one–fourth mile, turn left. The path meanders along the edge of the lava flow through mountain hemlocks, firs and pines. Take note of an unusual number of trees with knobby deformations, caricatures of their more normal companions. In less than a mile you'll come to a trail junction. Stay left on the PCT (the generally accepted direction is clockwise on this loop). A short distance later you'll notice a small unnamed lake on the left and soon after, a fine western white pine (these have the largest cones in our region except for a few scattered sugar pines).

The trail gains elevation steadily as it shelves along a cinder cone through a partly forested, partly treeless slope carpeted by ferns. Take your time going uphill; don't forget to breathe deeply and expel all your air. About 30 feet after you pass a downed mountain hemlock sectioned out for the trail, turn and look back. Sing the *Hallelujah Chorus* or just say *WOW*. Find Belknap Crater, Mt. Washington, Three Fingered Jack, Mt. Jefferson and Mt. Hood. Take a picture and continue. When you see a gulch of red cinders and chartreuse ground cover on the left, look for azure

North Matthieu below on the right. Blue lupine bloom here in summer. Follow the path across a black cinder slope to South Matthieu Lake, a sunny jewel between the cinder cones of Scott Pass.

When you're done feasting on the beauty — and perhaps lunch — go back to the nearby junction and follow the sign arrow toward North Matthieu. This fun little trail brings you quickly to another gorgeous lake that warrants some exploration. From North Matthieu, you'll switchback through a glorious forest of old–growth mountain hemlocks, subalpine firs and lodgepole pines — great patriarchs ruling their domain! After gawking, oohing and ahhing, look left to the lava flow edged by a pretty green glade. Watch for a small lake filled with "alligator" logs on the right. The path narrows to a deer trail through a peaceful meadow bordered by lava flow, then connects with the PCT. Go left through the caricature forest, watching for a right turn that takes you back to the parking area.

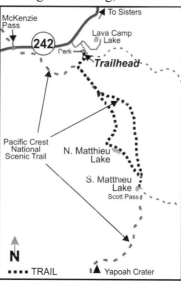

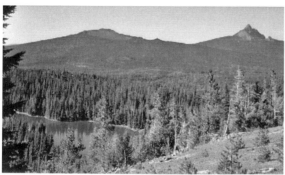

North Matthieu Lake

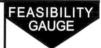
TRAIL CONDITION
mostly smooth, some roots & rocks

TRAILHEAD FACILITIES
outhouse at Lava Camp Lake

EXPOSURE
mostly shaded

USE
🚶 🐴
moderate

NOTES
Trekking poles helpful for short exposed slope; mosquitoes likely in mid-summer; camera a must!.

TIDBITS

The Pacific Crest Trail and the Appalachian Trail were the first national scenic trails named by Congress in the 1968 National Trails System Act. The PCT traverses the 3 wilderness areas of the DNF for nearly 100 miles: 40 in the Three Sisters, 17 in the Mt Washington and 36 in the Mt Jefferson Wilderness. Volunteers work over 400,000 hours annually on national trails.

HIKE

125

14 miles to Bend

Water
Geology
Forest
View

This magical outing rewards the hiker with great variety. You'll pass waterfalls, quiet pools and white water rapids. You'll see steep cliff banks, grassy shores and lava flows that changed the course of the river. You'll walk over an old railroad grade, along meadows of grass and willows, and through forests of massive pines and firs. Be sure to bring your camera; there are many "postcards" here.

Getting there

- *Drive 10 miles south from Bend on Highway 97.*
- *Turn right at the sign for Lava Lands Visitor Center.*
- *Turn left immediately and drive almost 4 miles to the Benham Falls picnic area.*

MILES
7.5

ELEV. GAIN
< 100'

PERMIT
NW Forest Pass

OPEN
April –
December

MAPS
Deschutes Nat-
ional Forest
Map, USGS
Benham Falls.

Walk toward the water to intersect the riverside trail. Go to the right (south) to a footbridge over the river. After crossing, follow the smooth former railroad grade along the Deschutes. This grade continues all the way to Benham Falls, but the hiking path diverts to the right just before the falls. Watch for ponderosa and lodgepole pines, and grand firs with their flat needle pattern, as well as a few small aspen trees plus plenty of bitterbrush and willows. Look also for views of Broken Top, South Sister and Lava Butte. You'll hear the thundering of the falls before you reach them. You might hear the roar of a freight train, too, as it grinds up the grade beyond the lava ridge on the river's far bank. The trail runs into a cedar–rail bordered footpath that switchbacks down to a viewpoint over Benham Falls, which is more a long series of cascades than a cliff drop. Even so, the rushing white water makes quite a dramatic sight as it swirls through the canyon.

Just a few steps back from the overlook, the hiking trail heads downriver. This scenic section follows the riverbank, sometimes at water level, sometimes high above. The lava flow is still visible above the far bank as are small groves of aspen trees, which turn brilliant gold in October. Anglers frequent this portion of the Deschutes, often wading, but occasionally using small boats. The trail leaves the river and winds through a mixed forest of aspens, pines and firs, then skirts a grass meadow bordered by willows. You'll come back to the river at Slough Camp, 1.5 miles from Benham Falls. Facilities here include an outhouse and picnic tables. Look for the trail marker near a boat ramp and continue north around a picturesque cattail pond. The path returns to the river, crosses large Ryan Ranch Meadow and passes through a gap in a fence. Continue to the picnic area and beyond to view Dillon Falls, another series of cascades. At the first drop, look for springs coming from the far lava bank to join the cascade. Walk downstream past several more scenic white water drops. The turnaround point is where log "steps" lead down to water level.

FEASIBILITY GAUGE

TRAIL CONDITION
mostly smooth

TRAILHEAD FACILITIES
outhouse, (also at Benham, Slough & Dillon)

EXPOSURE
mostly shaded

USE
🚶 🚲
moderate to heavy

NOTES
Trail can be muddy in spring; be prepared for mosquitoes in summer.

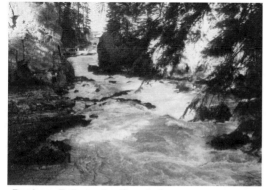

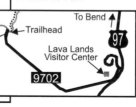

Benham Falls on the Deschutes

TIDBITS

James R. Benham moved to Deschutes County in 1879 and was one of five pupils to attend the first school in Bend. In 1885 he filed on a homestead near Benham Falls, which bears his name. The government rejected his claim, and he settled downstream nearer to Bend.

HIKE

F A C T FINDER

27 miles to Bend

Forest
View
Geology

This moderate outing puts you within 'wow' range of South Sister. Hemlock forest gives way to rolling plain surrounded by interesting geological features, including two snow peaks. Many of the cars in the parking lot will belong to peak climbers, so you may well have the trail mostly to yourself. Weekdays are best, however, as the lot will fill up on summer weekends.

Getting there

■ *Drive west from Bend on Century Drive/Highway 46 to the Devil's Lake sign (25.2 miles from the Century/Mt Washington/Reed Market circle).*
■ *Turn left into a parking area. The trailhead is located at the southwest edge of the parking lot. Fill out the free wilderness permit.*

MILES
6-7.5

ELEV. GAIN
600-1000'

PERMIT
NW Forest Pass

OPEN
July to October/ November

MAPS
Geo Graphics *Three Sisters Wilderness Map*, Deschutes National Forest Map, USGS South Sister.

Be sure to take the Elk–Devil's Lake Trail to the west and not the South Sister Trail which heads north. If you're on the right track, you'll shortly walk through a culvert under Highway 46. Gentle switchbacks lead you up a rock bluff and into the Three Sisters Wilderness. You'll curve left onto an old road that accessed a 1960's mining claim on Wickiup Plain. After a rocky stretch, the road becomes soft, sandy pumice. Walk through a lodgepole and hemlock forest that varies between airy and dark. At about ¾ mile, turn right at a sign for the Pacific Crest Trail. Walk another ¾ mile to a sign for Moraine Lake; keep to the right.

As the trees become smaller, watch for views of South Sister straight ahead. Soon the plain opens before you. Although it's dry and sandy, a number of wildflowers bloom here in July, including lupine, wooly pussy toes and dirty socks (the source of that pungent odor assaulting your senses). At the next junction, stay right to skirt the plain along Kaleetan Butte. Stay left at the Moraine Lake junction. Walk past a dramatic rock bluff toward LeConte Crater. Behind the crater, you'll notice at South Sister's base the broad Rock Mesa, a formidable deterrent to anyone wanting to climb the peak from this side.

Cross the plain and walk through two forest glades separated by a small meadow. As you emerge, you can see the Pacific Crest Trail across the way below House Rock and The Wife. Behind you, Broken Top and part of Bachelor are now visible. If you have the energy, the climb up LeConte will reward you with great views. Walk north and pick a diagonal route up the crater. When you've had your fill of this isolated playground, retrace your steps back to Devil's Lake.

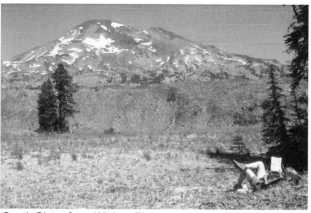

South Sister from Wickup Plain

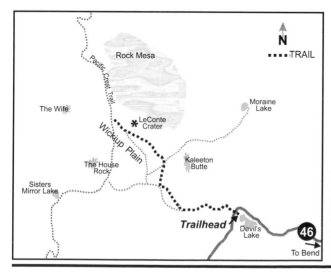

FACT FINDER

37 miles to Bend

Water
View
Forest
Geology

We include this enchanting hike because, in spite of the numbers of people who frequent the trail, it's one of our favorite outings. The numerous postcard views, generally reserved for more strenuous treks, make up for seeing a few people on the path. The trail becomes dusty in autumn, and you will appreciate trekking poles for several steep sections. We suggest you mentally prepare yourself for steep hiking by purposing to maintain an appropriate, if slow, pace and by keeping in mind the rewarding vistas. Our 78 year–old father thoroughly enjoyed this hike, in spite of the challenge.

Getting there

- *Drive south from Sisters on Road 16 (Elm Street), about 16 miles on a mostly paved road to a trail sign just north of Three Creek Lake.*
- *Turn right into the parking area along the Driftwood Campground road. Walk across Road 16 to the trailhead. Fill out the free wilderness permit.*

MILES 5 – 7

ELEV. GAIN 1200'

PERMIT NW Forest Pass

OPEN July/Aug to October/ November

MAPS
Geo Graphics
Three Sisters Wilderness Map,
Deschutes National Forest Map,
USGS *Broken Top.*

The trail starts up a steep slope through lodgepole pines, subalpine firs and mountain hemlocks. You'll gain almost half the elevation in the first three–fourths mile, but you'll appreciate a couple of short flat sections. Look often toward the west for stunning views of the Cascades and Three Creek Lake. A few openings in the forest also provide glimpses of the High Desert to the east. When you reach the edge of the rim, the trail levels out somewhat and passes the wilderness sign, continuing south for about one–half mile before turning to the west. As you walk another mile or so across the plateau, you'll gain more elevation and pass through two charming mini forests of stately hemlocks and firs. Look for views to the north of Mt. Washington and Three Fingered Jack, Mt. Jefferson and Mt. Hood. Rock hounds will enjoy all the variety and colors of rocks and formations along this segment of the route.

An unmarked trail to the right leads to the edge of a cliff overlooking Little Three Creek Lake and heart–shaped Three Creek Lake, surrounded by forest 1000 feet below. From this windy viewpoint at about 7700' you'll also witness a geologic wonderland, remnants of bygone volcanic activity. You might find shelter under a tree near the overlook to enjoy lunch. An optional extension continues from the main trail junction another mile or so to a viewpoint at nearly 8000 feet. There are several trail choices that lead to a small ridge–top plateau with lava bombs and gnarled trees. The northern–most trail winds partially along a narrow cinder shelf; those disliking exposure should avoid this path. The plateau offers a look at dramatic cliffs, as well as Broken Hand and Broken Top. When you've had your fill of this alpine magic, re-trace your steps back to the trail-head. Trekking poles help take some stress off the knees on the downhill stretches.

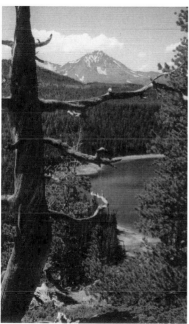

View to Three
Creek Lake and
North Sister

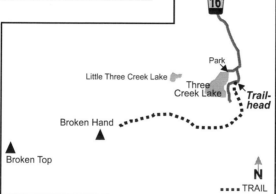

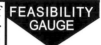
HIKE

44 miles to Bend

Water
Forest
View
Geology

If you're looking for a good workout and a chance to experience the Mt. Jefferson Wilderness, then this hike's for you. Carl Lake is an alpine oasis, not only beautiful, but swimmable if you don't mind cold water. Cabot Lake makes a pleasant rest stop. Mt. Jefferson is visible for much of the route. Trekking poles are nice to have on the steeper portions of trail.

 Getting there

- *Drive 12.3 miles west from Sisters on Highway 20 to a sign for Mt. Jefferson Wilderness Trailheads.*
- *Turn right (north) and follow Road 12 for 3.7 miles.*
- *Turn left onto Road 1230 and drive 8 miles or so to the Cabot Lake trailhead parking area (follow signs). Fill out the free wilderness permit.*

**MILES
*9.4***

**ELEV. GAIN
*1000'***

**PERMIT
*NW Forest Pass***

**OPEN
*July/Aug
to October/
November***

MAPS
Geo Graphics *Mt Jefferson Wilderness Map*, *Deschutes National Forest Map*, USGS *Marion Lake.*

The trail heads west through a varied forest of dead and live Douglas–firs, subalpine and grand firs, mountain hemlocks, whitebark and western white pines, and even a few ponderosa pines. You'll also see quite a bit of shrubby underbrush, some bear grass and manzanita. When you pass the Mt. Jefferson Wilderness sign, start watching for glimpses of Mt. Jefferson's peak through the trees to the right. Sugar Pine Ridge is visible across a canyon carrying Cabot Creek and a lava flow. After about one mile of hiking, you'll come to an unmarked viewpoint where the trail makes a sweeping left turn. Look for Mt. Jefferson to the north and patches of lava far below. The trail meanders another mile, with the canyon falling away to the right, sometimes gradually, sometimes more steeply (you're never right on the edge). Take a side trail, unmarked and easy to miss, down a steep, rocky slope to Cabot Lake, a green gem encircled by trees.

Continue on the main trail up a number of switchbacks that prevent the path from being too steep; unfortunately, they won't prevent you from breathing hard. Part way up this slope, Mt. Jefferson again becomes visible to the north. Soon after the trail levels out, you'll skirt around an unnamed lake, which is likely to be dry in September. Watch for three more small ponds, one on the left and 2 on the right. As views open to Sugar Pine Ridge, Forked Butte and North Cinder Peak, you'll know you're close to Carl Lake, a large turquoise oasis with a craggy rock backdrop. Lovely picnic sites abound, and a swim is not out of the question here. Take time to explore around the north shore (look for the narrow "dam" that holds the lake back from the steep valley below), before starting your return trip.

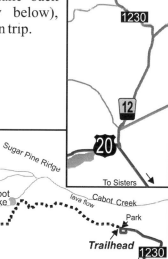

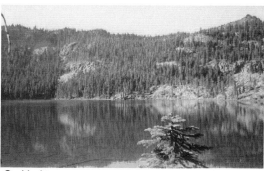

Carl Lake

TRAIL CONDITION
some roots & rocks

TRAILHEAD FACILITIES
none

EXPOSURE
shaded

USE
🚶 🐎
moderate

NOTES
Trekking poles helpful here; swimming optional.

TIDBITS

Mt Jefferson was named by Lewis and Clark in 1806 for President Jefferson. At 10,495', this andesite volcano with 5 glaciers is the 2nd highest peak in Oregon. The Mt Jefferson Wilderness Area, covering 109,092 acres, contains 150 lakes and 190 miles of trails. Timberland covers over 62% of its surface area.

HIKE

13 miles **to** Bend

NOTE
Access road is rough and narrow . Take high clearance vehicle if possible.

Forest
Geology
View

Getting there

MILES
< 2

ELEV. GAIN
< 50'

PERMIT
none

OPEN
April/May
to December

MAPS
Deschutes National Forest Map,
USGS *Benham Falls.*

Two unusual surprises await fit *Adventure Hikers* just a short distance south of Bend. Unfortunately, this outing is not appropriate for many mature folks. While fairly level, the hiking surface is just too rough. Boots and long pants are imperative; light–weight gloves are nice in case you have to steady yourself on the sharp lava. In spite of the negatives, we love this trek. It's isolated; it has pine trees older than your great–great–great–great grandfather. It has its very own dramatic "crack–in–the–ground." And, if you're lucky, it will treat you with that incomparable rumble — felt first, then heard, then seen — of a freight train pulling a grade! Tempting, isn't it! If you decide to take the challenge (not to say risk), don't say you weren't warned.

- Drive south from Bend on Highway 97 about 7 miles to the boundary sign for the Deschutes National Forest.
- At 0.7 miles past the sign, turn right onto an unpaved road.
- Drive about 300' north and turn back south at a Y.
- Continue south 1.5 miles, then turn west and drive 0.7 miles to Road 070.
- Drive 2.3 miles around Green Mountain and park in a small clearing (this is a very small parking area).

Walk the short distance from your car down to the railroad tracks on a faint unmarked path. Turn left (south) and follow the tracks for about one–fourth mile. Look closely for a small white sign on the right and what looks like a primitive road. The trail follows along this "road," which was begun in 1907 for an irrigation project. You'll pity those hapless pioneer road builders as you try to discern the least treacherous spot to place your foot. Several rock cairns along the path help guide you in the right direction. As you walk just under three–quarters mile through the rocky terrain, take time to enjoy the solitude and the eerie beauty of the lava "moonscape."

The approaching tree island, or *steptoe*, provides a pleasant change from the open black landscape. But tread carefully. Very near the northern edge of the island, a narrow crack in solid basalt gapes almost 50 feet deep and 10 feet wide. You'll enjoy exploring along the length of the crack before turning your attention to the wonderful ponderosa patriarchs around you. Fondly called *punkins* or *yellowbellies* by area pioneers, these oldsters have likely been guarding the lava flow for 300 to 500 years. When lava spilled from Lava Butte several thousand years ago, the flow diverted around this small rise, leaving enough fertile ground for the future forest.

Manzanita also seems to thrive here; if you come in spring you'll enjoy the small pink blossoms. We once waded through the shrubbery to the far side of the island, thinking a short trek over the lava would bring us to Benham Falls. That failed attempt made the "road" to the island look like a freeway. We hope you'll have the pleasure, as you head back, of experiencing the Burlington Northern freight train thunder by.

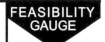
TRAIL CONDITION
rocky & rough

TRAILHEAD FACILITIES
none

EXPOSURE
open

USE

light

NOTES
Wear boots, long pants & sunscreen; for fit hikers only!

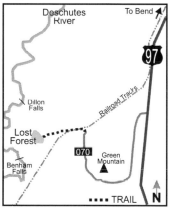

Deschutes River
To Bend
97
Railroad Tracks
Dillon Falls
Lost Forest
070
Green Mountain
Benham Falls
···· TRAIL
N

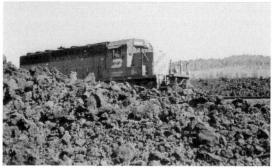

"Crack" on the steptoe

Train in the lava flow

TIDBITS
The flow you walk on here covers nine square miles and extends 30 to 100 feet deep. Two miles of railroad track were painstakingly laid across the lava in 1931 and are still used today by Burlington Northern.

HIKE

FACT FINDER

7 miles to Bend

Water Forest Geology

We love the raw beauty of this relatively new trail. Under construction for three years, the finished product does not provide a cushy journey, and many seniors will not want to tackle it. But those fit souls who go for it will enjoy the roar of the untamed creek and the feel of a wild frontier. If it weren't for a couple of homes across the creek on the high banks, you would swear you were pleasantly removed from any civilization.

Getting there

- *Drive west on Galveston Street, then Skyliner Road.*
- *From the Mt Washington Dr. Circle, drive 2.4 miles and turn right onto a dirt road. In just over 0.1 mile turn left on Road 4606.*
- *Drive 1.5 miles, cross Tumalo Creek and turn left into a parking area.*

MILES 4 - 8

ELEV. GAIN 150+'

PERMIT
none

OPEN
May-Nov.
can be muddy or snow-packed in spring

MAPS
USGS Shevlin Park, Deschutes National Forest Map.

Look for the trail to the left of the parking area. The steep, switch–back path gives a preview of the ruggedness of the trek ahead. This connecting spur intersects the canyon trail from Fremont Meadow in Shevlin Park. Turn left and walk along a ledge above Tumalo Creek. You'll see why horses and bicycles are prohibited here. While there are a couple of short stretches where you may feel slightly susceptible to slipping off the ledge, the main challenge comes from having to scramble over rocks. A nice, controlled pace and a trekking pole on your downhill side will give safety and confidence.

The forest progresses from mixed juniper and pine to mostly ponderosas and then a few big Douglas–firs (note the distinctive cones on the ground underneath). If you look closely, you may spot some tamarack trees, the only conifers that lose their needles in the fall. Manzanita, bitterbrush and snowbrush thrive along the early sections of trail. Oregon grape grows here, and if you walk in early June, you'll be treated to the beautiful purple blooms of shrubby penstemon. As you continue west through darker forest, watch for fern and balsam arrowroot with its yellow daisy–like flowers.

The most prominent features of this outing are the rushing creek down to the left and the rugged basalt cliff to the right. Should you get caught in a rain squall, you may choose to take shelter in one of the shallow caves or niches in the rock wall.

This is a perfect outing to custom tailor to your time and energy level on a given day. Turn around after 2 miles or when you reach the old Columbia Southern canal bed (which makes for an 8 mile hike). Or you could even take the Mrazek mountain bike trail back to the upper trailhead.

TRAIL
CONDITION
*very rocky
and rough*

TRAILHEAD
FACILITIES
none

EXPOSURE
*part open,
part shaded*

USE

light

NOTES

Trekking poles very helpful; this outing for fit, agile seniors only.

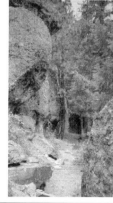

Magical path

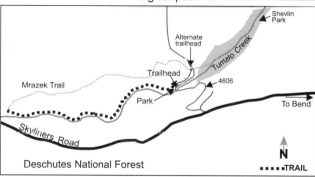

View of Tumalo Creek from the trail

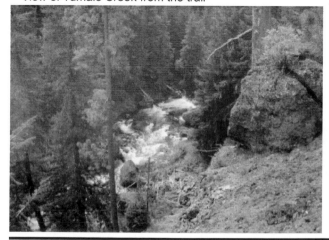

TIDBITS

Western junipers have been spreading in Oregon and now cover about 10% of the state's surface or 6.5 million acres. By sending their roots deep below the surface, they take water before it can reach other plants. Juniper is taking over grass-land and displacing native shrubs and even pines in Central Oregon.

HIKE

FACT FINDER	Climbers' Paradise

Smith Rock State Park is many things: a mecca for rock climbers, a highly accessible playground for hikers, and a visual feast for tourists and locals who don't want to expend much energy. The park is home to the area's most magnificent cliffs, some of which are visible from the parking area. *Hikers* and *Walkers* can utilize the map at the information board to customize their own outings. We've described a challenging, less–used trail for surefooted *Adventure Hikers* who don't mind a bit of scrambling. You'll definitely want trekking poles for this adventure. Winter is a good time to hike here; if you come in the summer, prepare for sun and heat and an occasional rattlesnake sighting.

26 miles to Bend

Geology
Water
View
Trees

Getting there

- *Drive north on Highway 97 through Redmond. From the north Y in Redmond, drive 5.4 miles to Terrebonne.*
- *Turn right on Wilcox Way, driving 2.6 miles to Crooked River Way.*
- *Turn left and drive 0.7 miles to Smith Rock State Park.*
- *Purchase the parking permit near the information board.*

MILES 6.3

ELEV. GAIN 1000'

PERMIT
state park pass

OPEN
all year

MAPS
Map at information board,
USGS *O'Neil.*

Walk west toward the canyon and follow a paved path along the rim. At a gate north of the picnic area, turn west and descend to the Crooked River. Cross the footbridge and turn right at the trail junction, following the river past an overhanging rock shelter and a giant ponderosa pine with spreading branches. The path curves to the east through a forest of junipers and pines and giant sagebrush. Look for caves and eagles' nests in the cliffs to the north. When you come to a weather guard station holding an emergency litter, take the trail to the left and switchback up to Burma Road. Walk left around the point where the canal tunnels into rock and follow the road to the southeast and then to the north, gaining elevation steadily until you're nearly 800' above the river. Most folks will want to take periodic breaks to catch their breath and enjoy the striking Cascade views to the west.

Near its high point, Burma Road turns west, then levels out before making a U–turn back to the northeast. Just before this U–turn, look for a path leading down to the left (west). At the next trail junction, stay to the right and contour around the north side of the ridge on a path that's sometimes faint and sometimes slippery with scree. Take note of the rock "fingers" and balancing rocks to the south and the canal and cultivated fields to the north. Grizzly Butte is visible to the northeast. The path turns south about three–fourths mile from Burma Road and continues along the western edge of the ridge. As you round a knoll, you'll come to a view of Monkey Face, one of the park formations popular with climbers. From this point, you'll need to bushwhack west and south around boulders (look for mountain mahogany here), down an unmarked route of loose dirt and scree. You'll soon come back to a visible trail that leads to the river, following it all the way back to the footbridge. This pleasant stretch, with just a few ups and downs, affords time to enjoy the river and study the cliffs dotted with climbers. Your adventure ends when you cross the bridge and climb the short, steep path back to the parking area.

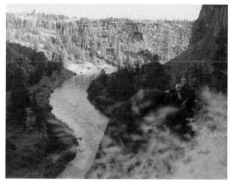

View of Crooked River

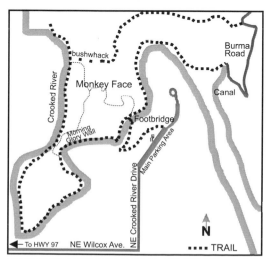

TRAIL CONDITION
mostly smooth, some rocky scrambling

TRAILHEAD FACILITIES
pit toilets, tables

EXPOSURE
open

USE
🚶🚲🐎
heavy

NOTES
Trekking poles a must; sun protection imperative; rock scramble; bring binoculars.

TIDBITS

Smith Rock State Park supports 400,000 visitors annually. Rock climbers from around the world are attracted to popular park formations with names like Monkey Face, Pleasure Palace, Wombat, Spiderman Buttress, Shipwreck and Picnic Lunch Wall.

HIKE

139

The Moonscape

37 miles to Bend

View

Geology

This challenging outing will please *Adventure Hikers* — it's the favorite area trek for one man we know. The geologic features make it unique in this guide. Those who love treeless hiking and far–reaching views will be amply rewarded. Trekking poles are strongly recommended. You will appreciate having sturdy hiking boots, not only on the lava, but also descending the steep, sandy Belknap cone. Less hardy *Hikers* might walk to Little Belknap and eliminate the scramble up Belknap. Wear sunscreen!

Getting there

- *Drive west from Sisters on McKenzie Highway 242. At McKenzie Pass, note Belknap Crater, the large rounded red cone to the north, and Little Belknap to the right. Also note two tree islands in the lava closer to the highway – you will walk around these islands.*
- *1/2 mile beyond the pass, turn right into a parking area.*

MILES 8.5

ELEV. GAIN 1800 '

PERMIT
NW Forest Pass

OPEN
July to October/ November

MAPS
Geo Graphics *Mt Washington Wilderness Map*, *Deschutes National Forest Map*, USGS *Mt Washington.*

Find the trailhead sign and walk down the sandy Pacific Crest Trail, which runs west briefly then passes around the east side of the first tree island, sometimes called a steptoe, and the west side of the second island. Look for lodgepole pines, subalpine firs, a few small mountain hemlocks, and even some ponderosa pines. After about three–fourths mile, you'll leave the trees behind and start the open trek through lava. This is like walking on very large, porous gravel. We felt it necessary to keep our eyes on the trail most of the time. You'll want to take many brief stops to look back at Black Crater, North and Middle Sister (with Collier Cone and Little Brother in their foreground), and at the fascinating lava formations all around you. Note the lack of vegetation with an occasional lone sapling or bush rooted in a pocket of soil.

As you approach the right turn to Little Belknap at about 2.4 miles from the trailhead, watch for views of Mt. Washington's rugged peak straight ahead. Walk past the Little Belknap trail (you'll hike this on the way back), and walk out of the lava flow through an open cinder field. Notice the trails on the bare south face of Belknap. You might want to come down this way, but we suggest going up on the north side. Continue walking a bit farther north then cut west through the stately mountain hemlock trees. Walk up a steep, bare section, then through scrubby whitebark pines past a small bowl. Watch for views of Mt. Jefferson to the north. Skirt around another minor crater, following the rim briefly west, then south, then back east. You'll see the main crater down to the south of this east rim. There are two "peaks," one with a small stacked rock shelter that makes a good lunch spot when the wind's not gusting. Take time to enjoy the 360–degree views. If you're up to a steep descent, go back west past the lesser "peak" and look for one of the trails leading east down the south face. These routes are fairly easy on the knees because they're so soft. Remember to lean back slightly and flex your knees for good balance.

On the return trip, take the detour to Little Belknap. The last stretch of trail snakes steeply through rocks and cinders to its peak. Note the three caves along the trail. The uppermost has a rimmed "crown" and a deep hole at its eastern end. You can actually scramble through the second tunnel–like cave with its smooth, shiny roof. As you walk back to your car, enjoy the mountain view, always keeping one eye on the rough trail. The jagged, smaller peak out to the west of the Sisters is The Husband.

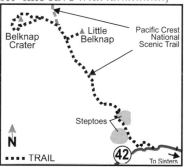

Belknap Crater from cave on Little Belknap

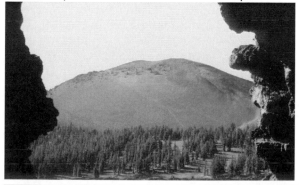

FEASIBILITY GAUGE

TRAIL
CONDITION
*rocky,
sandy*

TRAILHEAD
FACILITIES
*outhouse
(1/2mile east)*

EXPOSURE
open

USE
moderate

NOTES
Use trekking poles & hiking boots; wear sun protection.

TIDBITS
Belknap Crater is considered a fine example of a halocene shield volcano. Now extinct, the basalt cone erupted just 1400 years ago, slightly later than nearby cinder cones, Collier, Yapoah and Four-In-One. The Pacific Crest Trail skirts Belknap and Little Belknap on its 2650-mile route from Canada to Mexico.

HIKE

FACT FINDER

50 miles
to
Bend

Water
Forest
Meadow

As you hike toward an alpine gem in a meadow setting, it's fun to imagine how supplies were brought to this remote location for the log shelter by the lake. On the southwestern tip of our fifty–mile radius, the outing has a unique charm that's sure to draw you back in future summers. Several lovely lakes and some old–growth firs and hemlocks add to the adventure. This is a long outing for many *Hikers*, but there's not much elevation to gain. A swim in Cultus Lake might make a pleasant reward on the return trip.

Getting there

- *Drive west from Bend on Century Drive/Hwy 46 about 45 miles to the sign for Cultus Lake; turn right.*
- *Drive about 1 mile; turn left at a sign for Little Cultus Lake.*
- *Drive to a sign for Deer Lake Trailhead and turn right.*
- *Drive past trailhead all the way to Deer Lake (stay left at junctions) & park. The distance from the Little Cultus turnoff to Deer Lake is about 4.5 miles.*

MILES
10.2

ELEV. GAIN
200'

PERMIT
NW Forest Pass

OPEN
July to October/ November

MAPS
Geo Graphics *Three Sisters Wilderness Map*, Deschutes National Forest Map, USGS *Irish Mountain.*

Take the lake trail to the right (going counter–clockwise around lake). Walk to a junction and stay right (you can fill out a wilderness permit here or at the next entry point). Continue along the dusty trail through a varied forest of Englemann spruce trees, mountain hemlocks, subalpine and grand firs, lodgepole and western white pines. At about one mile from the junction, look for sparkling Cultus Lake through the trees. Follow along the edge of a lakeside campground accessed only by boat or trail. Soon you'll cross a creek flowing from Muskrat Lake on a wonderful, giant log bridge with handrail. You'll come to another view of Cultus Lake and then another trail junction. At this point three miles from Deer Lake, you'll enter the Wilderness. Fill out your permit, if you haven't already, and continue to the left toward Teddy, Muskrat and Winopee Lakes.

When you reach the sign for Teddy Lakes, stay left (save Teddy Lakes for the return trip). Continue 1.4 miles to Muskrat Lake. Watch for a green mini– meadow on the right and some grand mountain hemlocks in the denser section of forest. As you approach Muskrat, notice the green creek glade out to the left. As the creek widens into a still pool, look for bright green meadow grass through the trees. Shortly, an incredibly picturesque sight greets you — Muskrat Lake and a vintage log cabin. You'll want to visit the cabin and read the history tacked to the wall. A clearing in the woods beyond makes a nice spot for lunch.

Retrace your steps to the Teddy Lakes sign. This side trip will add 1.2 miles to the outing. Small Teddy is first on the left; large Teddy is a lovely alpine lake with a few Douglas–fir trees near the shore. Return to the sign, turn left and go back to Cultus Lake. Watch for a glimpses of Cultus Mountain during this section. Continue around the lake, stay left at the junction, and return to your car at Deer Lake.

Alternate directions: Instead of turning left to Little Cultus, drive to the end of the Cultus Lake campground and park at a trailhead. Walk around the lake to a junction with a sign for Winopee Lake; when you reach the wilderness entry point, fill out a permit and proceed as described above.

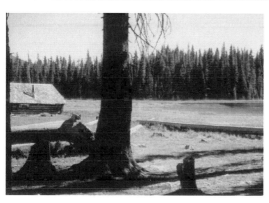

Muskrat Lake & cabin

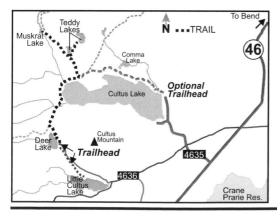

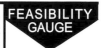

FEASIBILITY GAUGE

TRAIL CONDITION
some roots & logs

TRAILHEAD FACILITIES
outhouse (at nearby campgrounds)

EXPOSURE
airy forest

USE

moderate to heavy

NOTES

Mosquitoes likely in mid-summer; swimming optional.

TIDBITS

Many years ago, a young forest service worker was stalked by a cougar for several miles while hiking to a lookout tower on 6759' Cultus Mountain to report a fire. We saw large cat tracks on a recent hike in the area. We also saw a marten chasing a squirrel. Look for otters, osprey, deer, herons, eagles and beavers in the area.

HIKE

FACT FINDER

32 miles to Bend

Forest
Water
Meadow

This long but gentle outing offers two special jewels – a quiet meadow that you'll likely have all to yourself and a watery jewel that feels as if it's a million miles from anywhere. The forest here is typical of the East Cascades, and the small burned area is illustrative of the effects of forest fire. For a shorter outing (7 miles), turn around at Island Meadow and return the way you came.

Getting there

- *Drive west from Bend on the Century Drive/Highway 46 to the Elk Lake Resort sign.*
- *Turn right (instead of left to the resort) into a parking area. The trailhead is located at the southwest edge of the parking lot. Fill out the free wilderness permit.*

MILES
10 - 10.5

ELEV. GAIN
1650'

PERMIT
NW Forest Pass

OPEN
July to October/ November

MAPS
Geo Graphics *Three Sisters Wilderness Map*, Deschutes National Forest Map, USGS *Elk Lake.*

Walk west to the sign for Horse Lake. Look left for the easily–missed trail to Island Meadow. Follow this trail up a rise through a lodgepole pine forest sprinkled with mountain hemlocks and a few white pines (notice the large cones). When the trail levels out, look back for views of Bachelor, Broken Top and South Sister. You'll pass through a burned area where some mature trees have survived and much small vegetation has sprung to life. At the one mile mark, join the PCNST (Pacific Crest Trail) and immediately enter a shady moss–draped hemlock forest.   1.3 miles of walking brings you to a small lake on the left and a junction in a lovely little meadow. Continue straight on the PCNST about a mile through forest that now contains subalpine firs.   After crossing over a creek, you'll see Island Meadow through the trees and you'll have to step off the trail to the right to reach it. This makes a good spot for a food and photo break.

Go back to the trail and stay westward to a junction. You'll leave the PCNST now and turn north.   The signpost says "4337" and the DNF map says "3515." This forest includes beargrass and huckleberry as well as several mini–lakes near the path. Go past a trail to the left and turn left at the junction for Horse Lake. Pass another left–fork trail, then take the trail pointing to

Sisters Mirror Lake. Cross a good–sized creek on stepping stones and walk a few hundred feet, watching for Horse Lake through the trees to the left. A faint path leads down to the lake. For a nicer resting spot, continue on around the lake to the northwest side to a rocky bluff.

On the return trek, retrace your steps just to a left junction to Sisters Mirror Lake. Next, stay right at a sign for Elk Lake. This 3–mile forest trek is sprinkled with several grassy drainage areas. As you approach the parking area, the homemade ice cream at the Elk Lake store may call your name.

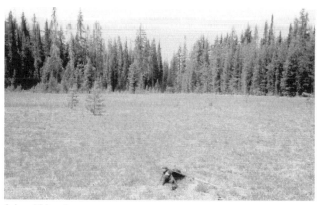

Island Meadow

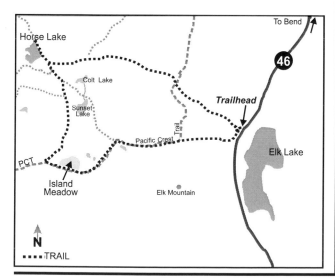

To Bend

N

····TRAIL

FEASIBILITY
GAUGE

TRAIL
CONDITION
*mostly smooth,
some roots
& rocks*

TRAILHEAD
FACILITIES
outhouse

EXPOSURE
airy forest

USE

light

NOTES
Mosquitoes are highly likely in mid-summer; watch for horse-packers on the upper section. Elevation gains are fairly gradual.

TIDBITS

The Cascade Lakes Highway is a USFS National Scenic Byway. The early wagon road was cleared by explorers Nathaniel Wyeth and John Fremont and replaced in 1920 by a road from Bend to Elk Lake. Currently the scenic route covers about 87 miles with a north entry point in Bend and a south entry point 3 miles north of LaPine.

HIKE

FACT FINDER

37 miles to Bend

View
Water
Forest
Meadow
Geology

This awesome outing is long for *Mature Hikers*, but it's well worth the effort. Pick a nice day, start early and take your time, bring plenty of food and water. You'll be rewarded with gorgeous meadows, hidden alpine lakes, and views to write home about. You will appreciate trekking poles on steeper parts of the route and, as on all long outings, you'll want to go prepared for weather changes and emergencies.

Getting there

- *Drive 14.3 miles south from Sisters on Road 16 (Elm Street) to a trail sign. Park on the left.*
- *Cross the road and walk up the berm to the trail which follows the old road to the original trailhead.*

In 2010 the USFS moved the trailhead out to Road 16 due to excessive wear on the old road. The walk to the former trailhead is 1 mi, making this trek 2 mi longer than it used to be.

MILES
13 – 15

ELEV. GAIN
1200 –1500'

PERMIT
NW Forest Pass

OPEN
*July/Aug
to October/
November*

MAPS
Geo Graphics
Three Sisters Wilderness Map,
Deschutes National Forest Map,
USGS *Broken Top.*

Follow the old road for a mile, then continue west on a wide, well-used trail through lodgepole pines, subalpine firs and mountain hemlocks. Bicyclers turn off onto the Metolius Windigo Trail, which you'll cross just before entering the Wilderness at rushing Snow Creek. Continue a mile and a half to a footbridge over white-ish Squaw Creek, flowing from a glacier on Broken Top through the town of Sisters to its mouth at the Deschutes River. Another mile brings you to Park Meadow with its islands of lodgepole pines and views of the Sisters and Broken Top. Skirt around the meadow to the right past a small pond and cross Park Creek on a flattened log. At the junction stay left on the Green Lakes Trail. Walk just over half a mile, up onto a ridge. After a quarter mile or so, when you glimpse Broken Top ahead, look for a rock cairn and a faint trail heading up a rise to the left. While much less traveled, this trail should remain visible as it winds through small meadows to Golden Lake's meadow basin surrounded by snow caps. Savor this isolated alpine oasis while resting or lunching.

If you're up for even better views and a rewarding adventure, cross the meadow (jump over narrow creeks), and head up the creek gulch to the west of the lake. Hiking boots and trekking poles are definite assets here on this steep, one–mile hike to an alpine gem that you'll first glimpse at eye level. Continue beyond the first lake to a smaller tarn — a superb vantage point for studying Broken Top's rugged crags. You'll want your camera on the return trip to Golden Lake; there are numerous postcards in every direction. The trek back to your car might seem long, but there is much beauty to distract you. We decided that we would reward our-selves with a cheese-burger at Bronco Billy's in Sisters, and this culinary vision energized our steps.

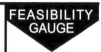

TIDBITS TIDBITS

Glacier views are a treat on this trek. Of the 17 in the Three Sisters Wilderness, look for Bend Glacier on Broken Top, Prouty on South Sister, Diller and Hayden on Middle Sister, and Thayer on North Sister. The Sisters are known as Faith, Hope and Charity, from North to South.

TRAIL CONDITION
partly smooth, some roots & rocks

TRAILHEAD FACILITIES
outhouse (Three Creek campground)

EXPOSURE
shaded & open

USE
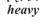
heavy

NOTES
Trekking poles & hiking boots an asset; pack for weather changes.

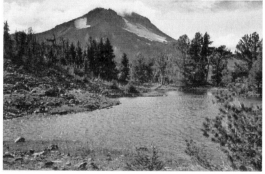

First unnamed lake above Golden Lake

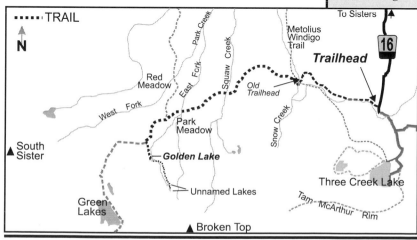

HIKE

147

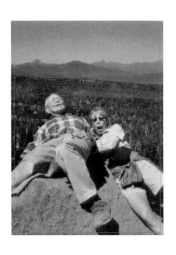

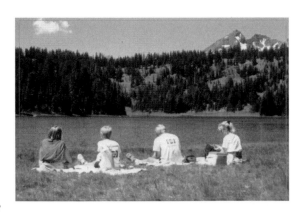

APPENDICES

Identifying and enjoying trees is to us one of the bonuses of hiking. We will attempt to simplify for you the task of identifying trees in the region. The first feature listed is the best identifier for mature trees. For more complete information, we recommend *Trees to Know in Oregon* (available at the Deschutes National Forest Headquarters in Bend), *National Audubon Society Field Guide to North American Trees, Western Region* and *Native Conifers of the Pacific Northwest* — a handy laminated tri–fold guide (both available through local bookstores).

On the outings in this book, the most typical forest contains lodgepole pines, mountain hemlocks and subalpine firs. A number of other trees make frequent or infrequent appearances.

PINE	*Slender needles grow in bundles; cones have thick, woody scales; grows in airy forests; has unique fragrance.*
lodgepole *2-needle bundles*	• ***Needles*** 2 per bundle, 1–3″ long • ***Bark*** dark, fine "alligator" grain, flaky • ***Cone*** 1–2″ egg-shaped, thick woody scales w/prickles *Only 2-needle pine in Oregon; slender & straight, growing to 100'; readily reseeds after fire; not many cones on ground.*
ponderosa *3-needle bundles*	• ***Needles*** 3 (rarely, 2) per bundle, 5–10″ long • ***Bark*** dark when young, rusty when mature; thick, ridged grain flakes off in "puzzle" pieces • ***Cone*** 3–5″ egg-shaped, thick woody scales w/prickles *Only 3-needle pine in Central Oregon; grows to 180'; some old growth stands; accounts for half the trees east of the Cascades.*
western white *big cone*	• ***Cone*** 5–12″ slender & often curved, thin scales • ***Needles*** 5 per bundle, 2–4″ long • ***Bark*** dark, fine "alligator" pattern *Grows to 180'; white lines on 2 sides of needles; only pine on these outings with cones this long.*
whitebark *contorted*	• ***Shape*** often contorted and under 50' tall • ***Needles*** 5 per bundle, 1–3″ long • ***Bark*** light gray and scaly, thin surface *1–3″ cones with thick, unprickled scales; white lines on all sides of needles; grows at treeline; each has own unique character.*
FIR	*Cones sit upright on branches, not many under tree; no woody pegs where needle joins twig; blunt (not prickly) needle tips.*
subalpine *needles massed atop twig, have white bloom*	• ***Shape*** "church-spire" crown; usually under 100' tall • ***Needles*** .5–1.5″ white line both sides, massed atop twig • ***Bark*** gray; smooth or ridged with resin blisters *2.5–4" purplish cones (cluster near top of tree); young twigs are greenish; grows at or near treeline.*

▪ *Needles*	.75–2″, shiny top, white underneath, point to side in 2 rows	grand
▪ *Bark*	gray–brown; thick ridged or smooth w/blisters	*shiny, flattened needles*
▪ *Size*	grows to 250′ with 6' trunk	
3–4" cylindrical green cones; shade-tolerant; likes moisture; grows at mid–elevations; round buds; interbreeds with white fir.		

▪ *Needles*	1.5–3″, white line or bloom on both surfaces; arranged in flat, V– or U–shape around twig	white
▪ *Bark*	gray; smooth with resin blisters or furrowed	*long needles*
▪ *Size*	grows to 200′ with 5′ trunk	
3–5" green, purple or yellow cones; grows in moist, rocky soils; young twigs are greenish; hybridizes with grand fir & hard to i.d.		

▪ *Cone*	3–4″ light brown with 3–pronged bracts	Douglas–fir
▪ *Bark*	red–brown, deeply furrowed & corky	*3-pronged bracts on cone*
▪ *Needles*	1″, green above, 2 white lines beneath	
▪ *Size*	can grow over 250′ west of Cascades	**NOT A TRUE FIR**
Not a true fir; cones hang down, unlike true firs; likes moisture; twigs orange when young with pointed buds; twigs droop.		

Cones hang down; woody pegs where needle joins twig; pointed (prickly) needle tips.	SPRUCE

▪*Needles*	.75–1″, spread around twig, sharp tip, 4–sided	Engelmann
▪ *Cone*	3–4″ light brown with ragged, papery scales	*sharp needles*
▪ *Bark*	purplish gray or brown with thin, loose scales	
Needles have smell of skunk when broken; usually less than 100' tall; likes cold, moist site; tolerates shade.		

Short needles; small cones that hang down; drooping tree top (leader) and branch tips.	HEMLOCK

▪*Needles*	<1″ bluish; massed around twig like starburst	mountain
▪ *Bark*	brown with ridges, deep furrows when mature	*starburst needle clusters*
▪ *Cone*	brown, 1–3" with rounded scales	
Grows to 100' with 3' diameter; mature trees easy to confuse with Doug-fir east of Cascades (look for cones to identify).		

Needles ("leaves") with overlapping scales; aromatic wood; reddish-brown bark that peels off in strips.	FALSE CEDAR

▪ *Cone*	1″ brown, duck–bill shape with 6 long scales	incense-cedar
▪ *Needles*	flat sprays of overlapping scales, flared at tip	*duck–bill Cone*
▪ *Bark*	rusty, stringy & flaky, somewhat furrowed	
Grows to 100' with 3' diameter; dense, matted foliage.		

▪ *Cone*	.75″ brown, 8–12 scales with rosebud shape	western redcedar
▪ *Needles*	lapped scale sprays, whitish "snakeskin" under	*rosebud cone*
▪ *Bark*	rusty; long, stringy, fibrous strips	
Cones grow upward on branches; trees have very broad bases; located on western edge of Central Oregon region.		

LARCH	*A conifer, but deciduous; needles tightly bundled in stout "barrel" pegs on older twigs (current–year twigs bear needles singly).*
western larch *bundles on raised pegs*	■ ***Needles*** 20–40 grow out of conspicuous woody pegs ■ ***Bark*** rusty, furrowed, flakes off in "puzzle" pieces ■ ***Appearance*** straight trunk, open crown, light green foliage that turns gold in autumn *Also called tamarack; loses needles in fall; cones are 1–2" with long bracts like whiskers extending beyond scales.*
JUNIPER	*Their "cones" look like berries and grow only on female trees; foliage can be needlelike or scalelike; has distinctive fragrance.*
western juniper *blue "berries"*	■ ***Needles*** scalelike and regular needles w/distinctive odor ■ ***Bark*** rusty, fibrous and thin ■ ***Appearance*** usually gnarled and irregular, but can be quite symmetrical; shorter than most conifers. *Female trees have blue "berries" with whitish bloom; dot of resin under each needle or scale.*
YEW	*"Cone" is a poisonous red "berry" with single seed; contains natural chemical called taxol.*
Pacific yew *flaky bark*	■ ***Bark*** purplish, thin & smooth with rusty papery flakes ■ ***Needles*** 1" dark green (light green underneath); margins roll under, flattened in two rows on twig ■ ***Appearance*** under 50'; irregular branches grow to light
LEAF TREES	*Deciduous.*
aspen *round green leaf*	■ ***Bark*** greenish white & smooth ■ ***Leaves*** 2–3" bright green; ovate or round with smooth edges; "dance" in the wind ■ ***Appearance*** under 80'; grows in moist locations

Other leaf trees seen occasionally in the region are cottonwood, alder and willow.

Don't be discouraged if you have trouble identifying trees in our region. We consider it a challenging and fun diversion, and we still get confused occasionally. In a thick, mature forest where you can't touch the foliage, look at bark and cones. Distinguish older Douglas–firs from mountain hemlocks by the droopy foliage and distinctive cones. Both have deeply furrowed bark — the hemlock bark might be darker and slightly more vertically ridged.

You will notice that two similar–sized fir trees growing side–by–side may have different bark, one smooth and one furrowed. This seems to be typical and just another challenge in the game. The trees we call grand firs might be white firs, since the two hybridize and take on the others' features. Young grand firs are easy to confuse with Doug–firs — look for rounded buds and upright cones on the grand fir.

Enjoy the game, but, mostly, enjoy the wonderful trees on these outings!

Bend, Oregon — Monthy Climate Summary for period of record, 1/1/1928 – 9/30/2005

	Jan	Feb	Mar	Apr	May	Jun	Jul	Aug	Sep	Oct	Nov	Dec	Annual
Average Max. Temperature (F)	40.6	45.3	51.1	57.9	65.5	72.7	82.1	81.1	73.8	63.0	49.2	41.9	60.3
Average Min. Temperature (F)	21.6	24.1	26.5	29.7	35.4	40.9	45.6	44.6	38.4	32.1	27.1	23.5	32.5
Average Total Precipitation (in.)	1.77	1.04	0.82	0.65	0.98	0.93	0.47	0.49	0.41	0.72	1.41	1.87	11.56
Average Total Snowfall (in.)	10.7	5.3	3.2	1.2	0.2	0.0	0.0	0.0	0.0	0.2	3.6	7.8	32.4
Average Snow Depth (in.)	2	1	0	0	0	0	0	0	0	0	0	1	0

The invigorating climate is one of Bend's greatest assets. Folks love the sunny days, low humidity and cool nights of the high desert.

SOURCE: *Western Regional Climate Center* wrcc@dri.edu

153

Often we find ourselves on outings with folks of varying fitness levels. Some are eager for a challenging hike while others, for whatever reason, want a shorter, less strenuous activity. In this section we've organized group itineraries with two or more outings departing from a common staging area where tables and an outhouse (and often drinking water) are available. A group may park at the staging area, and each person can choose an appropriate outing (or remain in the staging area with a good book). It should be pointed out that groups of more than 12 people are discouraged in the wilderness. If you take a large group on a wilderness trail, plan to break into smaller groups and stagger the start times.

Safety	Appoint a group leader and a sweeper. Select the most qualified person for carrying first aid supplies and administering any necessary first aid. Establish a plan of action, destinations, meeting points and times, finish time, etc.
Smith Rock *all year* $3 park permit for each car *Driving Directions -* *see Outing 5*	***Staging area***: Smith Rock State Park (pit toilets, tables, drinking water; Juniper Junction Store nearby) ***Easy Option***: Viewpoint – *Outing 5* in this guide (0.5+ miles) ***Moderate***: Walk along the river as far as you like ***Challenging***: *Outing 56* in guide (6.3 miles)
Newberry *Jun to Nov* NW Forest pass *Driving Directions -* *see Outing 11,8,30*	***Staging area***: Picnic area at Paulina Falls (tables, outhouse; nearby at Paulina Lake are drinking water, store & restaurant) ***Easy Option***: (1) falls viewpoints – *Outing 11* (0.4-1.7 mi.); (2) with short car shuttle, Obsidian Flow – *Outing 8* (0.8 mi.) ***Moderate***: car shuttle from staging area to *Outing 27* (2.4-3) ***Challenging***: *Outing 30 plus* continue around the lake (7.5)
River Trails *all year* *Driving Directions -* *see Outing 26*	***Staging area***: Sawyer Park (tables, outhouse, drinking water; ½ mile to Bend River Mall) ***Easy Option***: Walk along both sides of river in park ***Moderate***: *Outing 26* in this guide (2.6 miles) ***Challenging***: *Outing 26 plus* walk south to Mt Washington Drive (3.8 mi. R.T.) or to First Street Rapids (5.6 mi. R.T.)
Benham Falls *Apr to Dec* NW Forest Pass *Driving Directions -* *see Outing 50*	***Staging area***: Benham Falls Day Use Area (tables, outhouse) ***Easy Option***: (1) short interpretive trail; (2) walk to Benham Falls (about 1 mile round trip) ***Moderate***: *Outing 50 as far as Slough Camp* (4 miles R.T.) ***Challenging***: *Outing 50* to Dillon Falls (7.5 miles R.T.)
Green Lakes *Jun to Oct* NW Forest Pass *Driving Directions -* *see Outing 18*	***Staging area***: Green Lakes Trail parking area (outhouse) ***Easy Option***: Fall Creek Falls - *Outing 18* (1+ mile) ***Moderate***: Soda Creek Meadow – *Outing 31* (2.5 - 4.5 miles) ***Challenging***: *Outing 31* plus *Outing 18* (3.5 - 6+ miles); or hike the *Green Lakes Trail*, not in this guide (about 9 miles)

Staging area: Ray Atkeson parking area (outhouse, lakeside) ***Easy Option***: Ray Atkeson Viewpoint - *Outing 1 (*0.4 mile) ***Moderate***: Sparks Lake – *Outing 23* (1.2 -2.3 miles) ***Challenging***: *Outing 23 plus* car shuttle 2 miles to *Outing 31* at Green Lakes trailhead (4.8 - 6.8 miles)	**Sparks Lake** *Jun to Oct* NW Forest Pass *Driving Directions -* see Outing 1
Staging area: Wizard Falls Fish Hatchery (restrooms, drinking water, grassy areas) ***Easy Option***: (1) walk around hatchery and along river; (2) car shuttle to Head of Metolius – *Outing 3* (0.4 miles) ***Moderate***: Metolius South – *Outing 36* (5.4 miles) ***Challenging***: (1) Metolius North – *Outing 37* (6 miles); (2) *Outings 31 6& 37* (11.4 miles)	**Metolius River** *Apr to Dec* *Driving Directions -* see Outing 36
Staging area: Little Cultus Lake (outhouse, tables, drink- ing water, lakeshore) ***Easy Option***: (1) walk along north lakeshore; (2) walk trail to Deer Lake (4 miles R.T. on level trail) ***Moderate***: Walk to Cultus Lake (7 miles); or car shuttle to Deer Lake, then walk to Cultus (3 miles) ***Challenging***: *Outing 58* – *c*ar shuttle to Deer Lake and walk to Muskrat Lake (10.2 miles)	**Deer Lake** *Jun/Jul to Nov* NW Forest Pass *Driving Directions -* see Outing 58
Staging area: Jack Lake Campground (outhouse, tables) ***Easy Option***: Explore around Jack Lake ***Moderate***: Walk to waterfall near Wasco Lake junction – Trail # 4014, last section of *Outing 42* (3.1 miles) ***Challenging***: Canyon Creek Meadow – *Outing 42* (4.5 miles); optional extension to upper meadow (adds 1.4 miles) and to viewpoint (adds another 1.6 m) is quite steep	**Canyon Creek** *Jul to Nov* NW Forest Pass *Driving Directions -* see Outing 42
Staging area: Scott Lake Campground (outhouse, tables) ***Easy Option***: (1) explore around Scott Lake; (2) walk to Benson Lake – 1st part of *Outing 47* (2.8 miles) ***Moderate***: Tenas Lakes - *Outing 47* (5 miles) ***Challenging***: *Outing 47 plus* continue to Scott Mountain (8.2 miles and 600' additional elevation gain)	**Scott Lake** *Jul to Nov* NW Forest Pass *Driving Directions -* see Outing 47
Staging area: Shevlin Park (outhouse, tables) ***Easy Option***: Explore Aspen Meadow & along Tumalo Crk. ***Moderate***: Walk along the road to Red Tuff Gulch; turn right & walk to rim trail; turn right & walk back to road (about 2 m) ***Challenging***: Rim Trail – *Outing 45* (4.7 miles)	**Shevlin Park** *all year* *Driving Directions -* see Outing 45
Staging area: Village Green Park (restroom, tables), two blocks south on Elm. *Less active members of a group can* *spend several pleasant hours in the quaint town of Sisters (wal-* *king, shopping, eating), while others drive to outings west of* *town (#'s 2, 13, 17, 35, 36, 37, 38, 40, 42, 47, 48, 49, 53 & 57)* *and south of town(#'s 32, 52 & 60). City parks include* Creek- side *off Jefferson,* Village Green, Barclay *on Hwy 20 mid-town.*	**Sisters**

Here we list a few tricks — gained from personal experience, not scientific data — that keep us on the trail longer and keep us more comfortable. We also note a few tips gathered from our reading of more authoritative authors. We certainly can't guarantee that any of these tricks will help you, but we hope that one or two items will prove useful and beneficial.

Feet *Keep them happy!* Your two feet contain about 250,000 sweat glands and can excrete up to ½ pint of moisture each day.	Numero Uno – ***well–fitting shoes*** (please see page 15); break them in with short walks before embarking on a long hike. ***Socks*** – they must wick moisture; a proven practice calls for wearing thin polypropylene liner socks and thicker wool or blend outer socks (no cotton); this helps prevent blisters. ***Blisters*** – STOP when something is rubbing; remove the pebble, smooth out the sock wrinkle, or apply moleskin to hot spots. If a blister has started, apply Second Skin (gel product by Spenco, a must–have for first aid kits) and cover with tape. ***Comfort*** – cushioned inserts will be a help to some (as we age, we lose our natural foot padding). Regularly trim toenails straight across. On longer outings, remove shoes and socks at rest breaks (air–drying helps prevent blisters); soak feet a few minutes in cold water if possible (reduces any inflammation). ***Bunions*** – ah, the joys of aging; Marsha has gained relief from a pesky bunion by choosing boots with roomy toe boxes, using toe separators, and wearing a bunion regulator at night. ***Report*** prolonged pain or changes in the feet to a doctor; don't let a minor problem turn into a major one.
Knees	Conditioning and stretching are important (see pages 19,20). ***Stride*** – when going downhill don't overstride; go slowly and take short, smooth steps. ***Trekking poles*** – these can take much stress off the knees, especially on downhill stretches. ***Trick*** – Marsha puts elastic rings (stitch 5/8" waistband elastic into a circle that fits snugly around the knee) around her ankles and pulls them up to the knee cap when going down steep hills; they're like mini knee braces. ***Treatment*** – after a hike, we relieve knee pain with ibuprofen, MSM cream (see page 20) and cold packs. ***Supplements*** – many doctors are now prescribing healthy compounds (MSM, glucosamine, etc.) for joint problems.
Form	***Posture*** – stand erect, keep lower back flat and pelvis tucked directly under the spine; try to keep upper body relaxed. ***Breathing*** – breathe at a natural pace with your heart rate. ***Striding*** – maintain a natural stride (usually short steps rather than long); foot contact should be heel to toe on the ground; swing arms forward and back but not in front of you.
Body Consciousness	Listen to your body. Don't expect optimal performance on inadequate sleep or diet. Start slow and build. Know your limits. *Mature hikers don't have anything to prove!*

Deschutes National Forest   541/383-5300
1001 SW Emkay, Bend, 02;   www.fs.fed.us/r6/centraloregon
   Sisters Ranger District   541/549-7700
Crooked River National Grassland   541/416-6640
Lava Lands Visitor Center   541/593-2421
Bend Metro Park & Recreation District   541/389-7275
   www.bendparksandrec.org
Bureau of Land Management   541/416-6700
3050NE 3rd St, Prineville, OR 97754;   www.blm.gov/or/
Oregon State Parks   www.prd.state.or.us   541/388-6211
www.trails.com, www.gorp.com, www.llbean.com,
	Trail &
	Wilderness
	Info

Forest & Wilderness maps – Deschutes National Forest Headquarters (1645 Hwy 20 E, Bend 97701) and Sisters Ranger District (just north of Hwy 20, west end of Sisters) ***USGS maps*** – Bend Mapping & Blueprint Inc, 389-7440, G.I. Joes stores, www.trails.com, www.maptech.com ***Local maps*** – Bend Chamber (777NW Wall St.) 382-3221	Maps
Bend Chamber of Commerce (777NW Wall St.) 382-3221 www.bendchamber.org www.ci.bend.or.us www.visitbend.com www.insiders.com www.gorp .com www.ohwy.com/or	Area Info
Check out the many great outdoor stores in Bend & C.O. for expert help with products and fit (see yellow pages). ***Products for foot & leg health, shoes, etc.*** – www.walkerswarehouse.com, www.footsmart.com, www.thewalkingcompany.com ***Headwear*** – www.sundayafternoons.com, www.solumbra.com ***Miscellaneous*** – www.americanhiking.org www.northernmountain.com	Gear
www.elderhiker.com www.realage.com www.chw.healthlinkonline.com	Health & Fitness Tips
Tree Guides – *Trees to Know in Oregon* (at Deschutes National Forest Headquarters), *National Audubon Society Field* *Guide to North American Trees, Native Conifers of the* *Pacific Northwest.* **Trees, Wildflowers, Animal Tracks, Geology** – *National* *Audubon Society Field Guide to the Pacific Northwest*	Plants

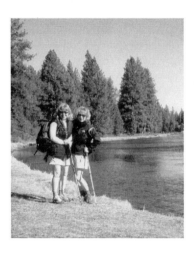

Sisters and native Texans, Johnson and Gray have hiked the West together for much of their adult lives. Johnson moved to Oregon in 1973. She raised two sons and now works in the advertising field. During the school year, Gray lives in Texas, where she works in school administration. She spends summers in Bend or in Lake City, Colorado.

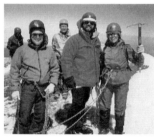

Gray at the top of Oregon

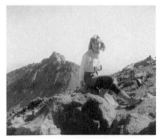

Johnson on Middle Sister